STRESS
PROTECTION PLAN

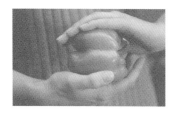

STRESS
PROTECTION PLAN

EVERYDAY WAYS
TO BEAT
STRESS AND
ENJOY LIFE

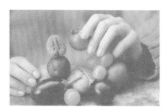

SUZANNAH OLIVIER

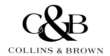

COLLINS & BROWN

To Lincoln Coutts, for teaching me to ask the right questions.

First published in Great Britain in 2000
by Collins & Brown Limited
London House
Great Eastern Wharf
Parkgate Road
London SW11 4NQ

Distributed in the United States and Canada by Sterling Publishing Co,
387 Park Avenue South, New York, NY 10016, USA

1 3 5 7 9 8 6 4 2

British Library Cataloguing-in-Publication Data:
A catalogue record for this book
is available from the British Library.

ISBN 1 85585 743 X

Editor: Fiona Corbridge
Designer: Sue Miller
Photography: Winfried Heinze and Matthew Dickens. See also
page 160

Reproduction by Classic Scan Ltd, Singapore
Printed and bound in Singapore

SAFETY NOTE: This book is written for those interested in nutrition
and its effects on health and lifestyle. Every effort has been made to
ensure that the contents are accurate and current, but medical and
nutritional knowledge are constantly advancing and this book is not
intended to replace expert medical advice and diagnosis. The author
and publisher cannot be held liable for any errors or omissions in
the book, or for any actions that may be taken as a consequence of
using it.

PUBLISHER'S NOTE: Great care has been taken to ensure that all
quotes have been correctly attributed. The Publishers apologize for
any unintentional errors or omissions and will correct such errors in
future editions.

CONTENTS

Introduction

Stress is nothing new; it was part of the lives of our prehistoric ancestors, and has continued throughout our evolution. But the type of stress we now experience has changed. We no longer, for the most part, have to worry about where we will sleep each night, how to keep warm, and where the next meal will come from. Our stresses have changed from those of survival to those of coping in a world that, to some of us, seems to have gone mad. Stress can come from many surprising quarters. Take information, for instance – we are used to thinking of information as a good thing, but today it is hurled at us from all angles, forming another source of stress.

It has been calculated that the average peasant living a rural existence in the eighteenth century was only exposed, during his or her entire lifetime, to the same amount of information that we would get in a single day's edition of the *New York Times*. Our modern world deluges us with a surfeit of information, and this can be very stressful. A typical office worker will fend off 65 communications in a single day – 35 phone calls, 12 pieces of mail, 18 e-mails... and this figure does not include junk mail, personal mail, or conversations with (and interruptions from) colleagues.

THE GRANDFATHER OF STRESS

In the 1930s, Hans Selyé did some pioneering work on stress. Selyé was a man of insight, but he was also rather clumsy. While making some investigations into a compound, which involved injecting it into his laboratory rats, the rats often escaped his grasp. Selyé had to chase them, often using a broom to shoo them out of corners. After a while, he noted that these unfortunate rats were getting peptic ulcers, that their immune system tissue (the thymus) had shrunk, and most interesting of all, that their adrenal glands (the glands responsible for the stress reaction) had enlarged. By a

process of elimination, and following further experiments, he concluded that stress was the cause of these changes.

Hans Selyé described the body's ability to overcome initial adversity and adapt to its new environment, or stressors, as "the General Adaptive Syndrome" (GAS). Selyé suggested that this adaptation, or stress response, was the body's way of maintaining its internal balance when faced with external imbalances. However, he noted that if the stressor continued for an excessive amount of time – the amount of time depended on the stressor and the person (or rat) experiencing the stress – then exhaustion would follow. The person would then become hypersensitive to the factor that triggered the stress reaction, and when faced with it again, would get stressed faster than before. Here are two examples of GAS:

● You are 12 years old, behind the school shed with your schoolfriends, trying out your first cigarette. You choke and splutter: this is your first reaction to the stress on your body. But you persevere, because it is "cool" to smoke. After ten cigarettes you can handle their effects – you have adapted (GAS). In fact, you have started to enjoy smoking, so you carry on for the next few decades. You get catarrh on your lungs and are more susceptible to colds and bronchitis in the winter (and eventually you could end up with emphysema or lung cancer). But then you give up smoking. You become oversensitive to cigarette smoke, and are now a born-again anti-smoking advocate, who walks out of the room if someone lights up.

● Your new boss decides that budgetary savings need to be made and fires a couple of people in the company. This soon has repercussions for you, because your workload increases. Now you have to handle the same amount of business as before, but without the assistance of two support staff. You are forced to adapt to this change, and start working late and at weekends to keep on top of it all. This has the inevitable consequence of ensuring that your social life goes to the wall. After a couple of years of this regime, you are exhausted, suffering regular bouts of illness, wracked by anxiety and prone to depression. Finally, you just

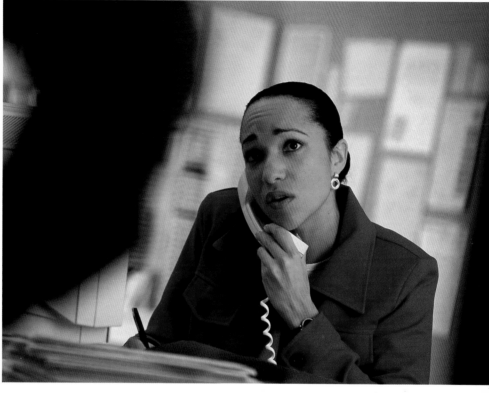

A change in responsibilities at work is likely to bump up your stress levels.

can't take any more, and quit your job. A complete life change follows, as you sell up your house and opt for running a small bar in a holiday resort. The final stage of the GAS is that you have now become oversensitive to the stressor, and never want to work in an office again!

If you have built castles in the air, your work need not be lost; that is where they should be. Now put the foundations under them.

HENRY DAVID THOMAS

CHAPTER ONE

who, me? stressed?

Feeling tense? Learn how to recognize the signs of stress

What is stress?

We are all aware that one person's stress is another person's excitement. To me, the idea of making a free-fall parachute jump out of an aeroplane, where I would have to rely upon one little cord pulled at the right moment, and one emergency back-up parachute (which may or may not work), is nightmarish. I find it hard to think of many things that would induce greater stress. And yet I have just received a photograph of a friend happily doing a charity jump, and having the time of his life. So what is stress exactly?

STRESS

The truth is that to be alive is to be under a certain amount of stress – it is an occupational hazard of living. Hans Selyé recognized this when he coined the phrase "eustress", meaning benign, or even beneficial, stress.

One example of this is the mechanism by which we wake up in the morning. Light causes the levels of adrenal hormones in our bodies to rise in the hour before we are due to wake up, even if it is dark outside. This prepares our bodies for action. One adrenal hormone, adrenaline, is also used for motivation and concentration – we set ourselves targets that need to be met, whether it is collecting the children from school or delivering a thesis. On the first night of a play, an actor's elevated adrenaline level gets him on to the stage and ensures a great performance – and, even months into a play's run, the same level of adrenaline continues to be produced. An athlete would be lost without the adrenaline that spurs her on to competing and focusing on winning. How often have you read interviews with high flyers who say that they thrive on the adrenaline rush generated by the cut and thrust of their job? Are their bodies under undue stress? Probably not.

"DIS-STRESS"

Stress is actually "dis-stress". Distress usually implies conflict, meaning that we are subject to a force that is the opposite of what we desire. The conflicts that can cause stress are many, and I am sure that you can think of endless examples in your life. For instance:

● You have to give a presentation as a part of your job, but you hate public speaking.

● You feel that you need a bit of a break, but have to look after your children.

● You want to try for a new job, but fear that it may not work out and you'll be worse off than you are now.

● You have agreed to do something for a demanding friend or relative, but it has disrupted your plans and you wish you had the ability to say "no" more often.

● You need to complete a project, but do not have enough time to do it.

All these situations are conflicts that require resolving before they wear you down!

The other major area of distress in our lives is a feeling of lack of control. For example, most people would assume that senior executives top the charts on stress scores. Yet blue-

If you feel that you are at the mercy of the whims of the world, and that other people control your life, you are likely to be under considerable stress.

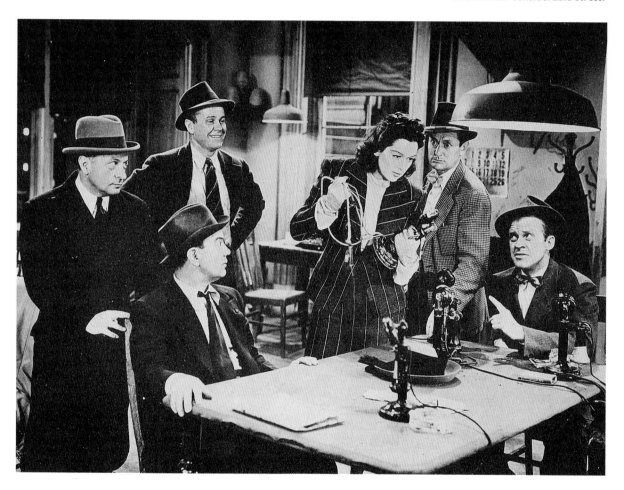

collar workers actually score much higher on the stress indices. It has been determined that this is because they do not feel that they are in control of their destiny in matters such as wages, working hours, type of work, who they work for and, ultimately, the ability to retain their jobs. One study found that fighter-pilots returning from war zones had considerably fewer stress problems than their crew, who had no control over what was happening.

Stress does not respect cultural, social or financial divides – everybody has some stress to contend with in their lives, whether it comes from work, family, money problems or another source. But some people cope with these external stresses better than others, and their stress-busting skills enable them to pick themselves up and get on with their lives. We will be looking at how you can acquire these skills and protect yourself from the effects of stress.

Stress from all angles

Stress, or "dis-stress", is very personal. But stress is not just a series of events that happens to us, or even our reactions to those stresses. Stress can be defined as anything that adversely affects the health or functioning of the body, such as injury, disease, depression or worry. These stresses on the body can come from many different directions.

MENTAL AND EMOTIONAL STRESS

We all have different stress triggers. For instance, consider the scenario where you are kept waiting for an appointment. Some people would pace up and down, looking at their watches, fuming at the indignity of being kept waiting and wishing that people could be on time. Some would use the time profitably by making notes for a project that they had been meaning to tackle for ages. Others would just let their mind wander, happy that they had some spare time to relax. Which person do you think is under more stress – or dis-stress? Who is feeling conflict and lack of control and who is not? Who is pushing himself mentally and emotionally?

PHYSICAL STRESS

Physical stress is not to be underestimated. For example, a reasonable level of exercise is good for us, but if we over-train, the body's reserves are put under stress and we make ourselves more susceptible to tiredness and illness.

When the body is wounded, a host of mechanisms jump into action to repair the damage. But if it is already overstressed, repair cannot happen efficiently. Inflammation may occur, which is an added stress for the body to cope with. Various health problems occur as a result of inflammation, such as asthma, eczema, psoriasis, irritable bowel syndrome, colitis, gastritis and arthritis.

ENVIRONMENTAL STRESS

We are surrounded by chemicals. Thousands of new chemicals have been introduced into our environment during the last 50 years. Man-made substances are found in food, water, cosmetics, household cleaners and garden products. The whole of this chemical load has to be dealt with by the body, specifically by the liver, which has to process, detoxify and store or eliminate the chemicals. Given that the liver also has a whole host of other jobs to do, such as metabolizing food, manufacturing proteins and processing hormones, it is not surprising that this increased workload causes things to go wrong. The system begins, slowly and imperceptibly, to break down: you feel below par, and this is followed closely by illness. Feeling low is enough in itself to compound mental and emotional stress.

NUTRITIONAL STRESS

Foods that do not agree with us (on any level) create a crisis for the body. These may be foods that overstimulate us, to which we are addicted, or which cause intolerance reactions. Minor nutritional stressors can be dealt with without too much trouble. As we have already seen, we have a tremendous ability to adapt. But if minor dietary stresses continue for too long, or if we slide into overusing major dietary stressors, then there is usually a price to pay. Another important nutritional stress factor is when the number of nutrients being absorbed from the diet is insufficient to maintain a healthy metabolism. This can occur for a number of reasons:

● The food itself may be low in nutrients because it has been over-processed.

● The variety of foods in the diet may be poor.

● Food and drink may come with other components, or pollutants, which impair the body's uptake of nutrients.

● Digestion may be impaired.

THE IMPORTANCE OF GOOD NUTRITION

Your diet can substantially influence your tolerance of, and response to, stress. Good nutrition, with a helping hand from natural supplements when necessary, cannot remove stress from your life, but it can help to increase your tolerance to it. It will temper the adverse effects of stress, and reduce the chance of long-term degenerative diseases associated with chronic stress. Alongside this, you can help yourself by limiting your exposure to a significant number of environmental stressors. Food also has a therapeutic effect and can help to raise mood and energy levels, helping to flip you out of a downward emotional spiral.

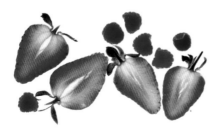

TOP FIVE ENERGY FIXES

1 Avoid all stimulants for a week and feel the difference. Ban sugar, chocolate, tea, coffee, alcohol and cigarettes. Go on, you can do it!

2 Eat a high-energy breakfast every day – wholegrain cereal, live yoghurt, sliced fruit and apple juice. Try wholegrain toast, almond nut butter and sliced strawberries. Make porridge with blueberries and soya milk. Squeeze fresh orange juice to drink.

3 Snack little and often on energy "givers" rather than "drainers". Choose fruit, live yoghurt, rye crackers, oatcakes, and vegetable sticks with bean dips.

4 When you are feeling lethargic, instead of slumping in front of the television with its energy-draining electromagnetic field (EMF), go for a walk to wake youself up. Increase the distance each time.

5 Get into the habit of pausing to take 20 deep breaths. Do it while sitting down, ten times a day. Fill your lungs with energy-giving oxygen. In Chinese medicine, an invisible life-force energy called qi circulates throughout the body. It is acquired by your first intake of breath as a newborn baby, and replenished by breathing.

We are promoted to the level of our incompetence.

Understand the level you are happy at.

ANON

Life events

Yet another way of analyzing stress and its results divides it into external stresses (those that happen to you) and internal stresses (those that you create for yourself). Below is a list of the most common major life event stresses, or external stresses. The list is based on the most frequently used assessment scale, the Social Readjustment Rating Scale. See how you score.

This is not a definitive list, as stress can vary according to circumstances. It is hard to decide whether some life events are "good" or "bad" stresses. For example, moving house involves a lot of upheaval and additional expense; on the other hand there is all the fun of making a new nest. Or the move may be because of reduced finances or a broken relationship. A "change in eating habits" also features on this list, which is ironic because making positive changes to eating habits is one of the most important ways of reducing the overall stress load on the body!

MINOR STRESSES

Studies have shown that by analysing your accumulated everyday trials and tribulations, you may gain a more accurate indicator of your risk of suffering a stress-induced illness than by examining the major stresses you have been subjected to.

Score 1 point for each factor that is affecting you.

❑ Partner starts/ stops employment
❑ Begin/end school, college, university
❑ Change in living conditions
❑ Moving house
❑ Change in religious habits
❑ Taking out a small loan
❑ Change in the number of family reunions

❑ Change in eating habits
❑ Minor law-breaking
❑ Trouble with the boss
❑ Change in work hours
❑ Revision of personal habits
❑ Changing schools
❑ Change in social activities
❑ Change in sleeping habits
❑ Vacation
❑ Christmas

Total score for this section...

■ If your score in this section is 5 or more, then add another 3 points for cumulative stress. Your new score is.............................

**A readjustment to your business
may well affect your wellbeing.**

MEDIUM STRESSES

Memorable life events, both pleasurable as well as
unhappy, can have an impact on your health. For example,
the risk of depression can be increased 1,300 per cent by
events such as separation or divorce, but also by stresses
that many people would imagine to be happy events, such
as starting college or having a baby.

Score 2 points for each factor that is affecting you.

❏ Pregnancy

❏ Sexual problems

❏ Business readjustment

❏ Death of a close friend

❏ Increase in number of marital rows

❏ Change in responsibilities at work

❏ Outstanding personal achievement

❏ Change in a relative's health

❏ New family member

❏ Change in finances

❏ Change to a new type of job

❏ Taking out a large loan

❏ A child leaves home

❏ Trouble with in-laws

Total score for this section...

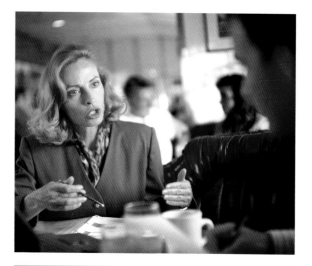

MAJOR STRESSES

Major stresses are connected with feelings of helplessness,
and include war, a relative's death, or personal injury.

Score 3 points for each factor that is affecting you.

❏ Death of a spouse/partner

❏ Divorce

❏ Marital separation

❏ Marital reconciliation

❏ Jail sentence

❏ Mortgage foreclosure

❏ Death of a close relative

❏ Personal injury or illness

❏ Marriage

❏ Retirement

❏ Being fired

Total score for this section...

■ Now carry the three scores forward to "Interpreting Your
Answers" on page 17.

Internal stresses

It is not only important to take life events into consideration when assessing your stress load, but also the way in which you handle these stresses. One scientist, after conducting trials on rats with different genetic "natures" or personality profiles, was quoted as saying that "the laid-back rodents suffer different diseases from the jumpy ones". This is mirrored in humans, and the way we react to stress can affect our health on many levels. Look at the following questions and answer "never", "rarely", "sometimes", "often" or "always".

	never	rarely	sometimes	often	always
Life factors					
Do you feel unhappy in your job?					
Is your domestic life unsettled?					
Do you consider yourself to be under stress?					
Are you discontented in your key relationships (such as with partner, parent or child)?					
Do you feel you are unhappy about other aspects of your life?					
Behavioural factors					
Do you internalize your problems and have trouble discussing them?					
Do you have a persistent need for achievement?					
Are you unclear about your goals in life?					
Do you easily become angry or irritable?					

	never	rarely	sometimes	often	always
Do you do two or three tasks at the same time, or find it hard to finish a task before starting others?					
Do you find it difficult to make decisions?					
Do you suffer from depression, or have you in the past?					
Do you have mood swings, get irritable, or become apathetic?					
Do you have any compulsive behavioural traits?					
Do you find it difficult to concentrate?					
Do you feel unable to cope?					
Do you feel you want to cry at the smallest problem?					
Do you have a lack of interest in doing things after work?					

Physical symptoms	never	rarely	sometimes	often	always
Is your appetite poor?					
Do you crave food when under pressure?					
Do you have addictions?					
Is it hard to sleep?					
Do you wake up tired?					
Are you susceptible to headaches or migraines?					
Do you get stress-induced indigestion or irritable bowel syndrome?					
Do you get stress-induced muscle tension?					
Do you get breathless or have palpitations without much physical exertion?					
Do you get dizzy?					
Do you have skin trouble – hives, rashes or eczema?					
Do you have less energy than you used to?					
Total the score for each column. Carry your scores over to "Interpreting your answers" below.					

INTERPRETING YOUR ANSWERS

Scoring external stresses, pages 14–15

What was your total score for Minor stresses? ....

What was your total score for Medium stresses? ....

What was your total score for Major stresses? ....

Your total score for this section: .... (a)

Scoring internal stresses, opposite and above

Score 0 for each "never" ....

Score 1 for each "rarely" ....

Score 2 for each "sometimes" ....

Score 3 for each "often" ....

Score 4 for each "always"..

Your total score for this section: .... (b)

Now add (a) and(b) together to get your overall score.

If your overall score is 0–20

You have a relaxed attitude which will help to protect you from the worst that life throws at you. Either you are naturally able to take things in your stride, or you have learned that stress begets stress. Keep up the good work, and eat healthily to support your positive mental attitude.

If your overall score is 21–40

Your life is under reasonable control, but you lose your grip from time to time and feel under pressure. If this is allowed to continue you may soon begin to experience minor health problems such as disturbed sleep patterns, indigestion, frequent colds and infections, and poor wound healing. Use the plans in this book to protect yourself from the effects of stress and to stay feeling in control.

If your overall score is 41–55

Pressure has been building up for a while, although it may not have had a detrimental effect on your health yet. It is time to reassess your life. Spend more time doing what you enjoy, and less time under pressure. The plans in this book show you how to fight stress. Incorporate the information into your daily life, and you should feel healthier and happier.

If your overall score is 55+

You are probably finding life a real struggle and need to get balance back into your life. If you are under a lot of stress you may find that you benefit from a support group or counselling. It is extremely important that you devise a strategy to help you to get back on track – use the plans at the back of this book. If a long-term plan seems too daunting, start slowly by devoting a weekend to pampering yourself first, and see how much you benefit. Then move on to a week-long plan, and finally to a month-long plan.

Mind matters

Everybody feels low from time to time. This is normal and it would be a bit odd if we were not sad, for instance, on hearing of the death or illness of someone close to us, or if we did not feel uneasy about a dramatic change in our circumstances. Feeling low can even be viewed as a part of the healing process – a time of reflection and introspection. But many people find that this natural tendency gets out of hand and impacts on their daily life. It can take different forms – lack of concentration, loss of sexual desire, anxiety, apathy, despair, depression or insomnia.

The genetic make-up of some people makes them more likely to suffer from depression than others (we will talk about ways to deal with this later). Feelings of gloom may even follow a seasonal pattern, known as SAD (seasonal affective disorder), which is when people feel much worse during the winter months than in the summer, because their exposure to natural light is lessened.

LEARNED HELPLESSNESS

One way of adapting to stress is to become apathetic and "helpless". It is a means of coping where you convince yourself that you can do nothing to alter the relevant circumstances, so it is not worth bothering to try. One study of rats revealed a lot about this learned helplessness. Rats in a divided cage were given a mild electrical stimulus through the floor on one side of the divide. They all ran to the other side for safety. When the divide was closed off, there was no escape route and they became resigned to their fate. When the door was reopened they did not try to escape again, even though they could see the open door. The symptoms of learned helplessness are easy to recognize in humans. After a failed exam, job interview or relationship, we can be overcome by self-doubt, questioning our abilities and wondering if we will ever succeed. Many people recover by working even harder to attain the desired result, but a significant number fall back on learned helplessness, and it may even become a feature of their personality.

POSTURE AND MOOD

It is very difficult to feel sad if you walk tall. Unhappiness is often reflected in poor posture, with drooping shoulders and a shuffling walk. Next time you catch yourself doing this, shift to walking briskly and hold yourself erect. Fix your eyes on a point high up, for instance the top of the trees or

Trying to make the unworkable work – doesn't work.

ANON

rooftops, throw your shoulders back and smile. Your whole mood will change immediately.

THRIVING VERSUS COPING

Thriving means enjoying yourself: living for the moment, maximizing opportunities, and making any given situation work to your advantage. The dictionary defines it as "to prosper, to flourish, to grow rich". Coping just means getting by, and dealing with situations or problems as they arise. Copers are people who shrug on a Monday and say, "Oh well, only five days until the weekend." This does not reflect a positive outlook to life, and I much prefer the idea of thriving rather than just coping.

There are many words that we use daily to describe what is going on and how we feel about it. Our choice of words defines how we see our world. Improving our outlook means eliminating some words from our vocabulary – one of them

ARE YOU SUFFERING FROM SAD (SEASONAL AFFECTIVE DISORDER)?

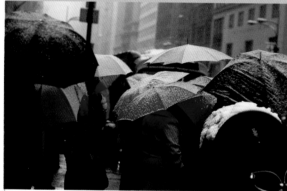

Most of us feel less sprightly in winter because it is cold, it gets dark early, and we suffer from colds and coughs more frequently. But for some people, these effects are magnified. They find the winter months really incapacitating, and may get quite depressed. If you feel that you come into this category, what can you do to help yourself at this low point?

1 One of the most favoured forms of treatment is a light-box. This is a bright light that simulates natural daylight. The treatment programme involves exposing yourself to the light for a period each day.

2 A diet high in sugar, alcohol and white flour products makes susceptible people more prone to feeling bad at this time.

3 Simulate a summer diet. Prepare for winter by freezing large quantities of summer berries, or buy them canned in natural juices. They are high in nutrients.

4 The herb St. John's wort has been found to be successful at relieving the depression associated with the winter months. Do not use it in conjunction with a light-box, as the herb causes photosensitivity (makes your skin sensitive to light).

5 If all else fails, shift your longest vacation to the winter, when you probably need it most. If possible, spend it in a sunny climate!

is "coping". Next time you are asked how you are responding to a problem, avoid saying "I'm coping with it" and switch to "I am dealing with it".

Other words, such as "I'll try", almost always doom attempts at change to failure, implying lack of action or a lack of success. Close your eyes for a moment and visualize yourself pushing a wall down. What did you see in your mind's eye? Most people picture the wall toppling to the ground. Now close your eyes again. Imagine that you are *trying* to push the wall down. What did you see? Most people envision a great deal of effort, which does not necessarily bring about a successful result. Strike the word "try" from your vocabulary, substituting the positive "I will do..." for the ineffectual "I will try to do...".

The final word to banish from your vocabulary, especially when you are talking to yourself, is the word "should". Think how many times you hear or use phrases that include the demon word. "You should to do this", "You should to do that", "You should deal with the stress in your life", "You should lose weight", "You should get more rest". It has unpleasant overtones of an overbearing person speaking to a smaller, weaker person. A lady I know had a wonderful sign in her office. Prominently displayed in large lettering, it read, "THOU SHALT NOT *SHOULD* ALL OVER THYSELF".

By getting rid of the three words "coping", "try" and "should", your life will improve. Discover how much better you can communicate, not only with others, but most importantly of all, with yourself.

THE FOUR-MINUTE MILE

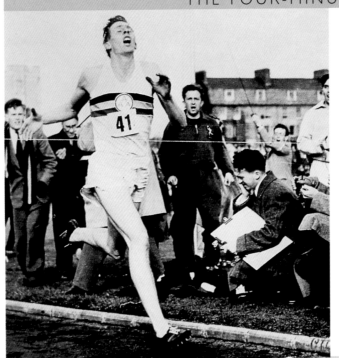

In the 1950s, Roger Bannister became the first man to run the four-minute mile. He managed to break a record that had been the pinnacle of man's running ambitions since the days of the gladiators. In the year following this great feat, more than 30 men managed to replicate his achievement. After two thousand years of striving, suddenly not one man, but several, managed to run the distance in less than four minutes. What changed? Did a new superbreed of runners suddenly appear on the planet? Was a great new training technique discovered? Neither of these things happened – the only change was that people went from believing that the record could not be broken, to believing that it could. Belief is everything. People could imagine themselves doing the same thing – they could see victory in their mind's eye.

BREAKING PATTERNS

One of the reasons we sag into learned helplessness is a little voice in our heads that confirms all our worst fears: "I knew I wouldn't get the job", "No one will ever like me", and so on. You need to silence that little voice for good, so next time something doesn't work out, respond in a way that is radically different to your usual reaction. This will change your mood and focus. We often do it automatically – for instance by pinning up cartoons over our desk, or firing off jokey e-mails Now, however, do it when you are feeling low. Here are some ideas to help you lighten up:

● Wear bright, sunny clothes in the middle of winter – see how many people comment!

● Throw a "newly divorced" party. Or a "newly sacked" party. Or an "I've got an overdraft" party (get everyone else to bring the wine).

● Keep some Mickey Mouse ears in your office drawer and wear them every time you are on the phone to a difficult client.

Our life is the creation of our mind.

BUDDHA

HOW TO TALK YOURSELF INTO HEALTH OR ILLNESS

BEING POSITIVE	BEING NEGATIVE
I eat healthily	I am going on a diet
I take full responsibility	It isn't my fault
I do not want to	I can't
Next time	If only
I can learn from this	It's a disaster
This is an opportunity	This is a problem
I can	I should
I feel confident	I feel guilty
I am flexible	I am disappointed
I am loved and appreciated	I am angry and frightened
I feel vital	I feel overwhelmed
I feel great	I feel OK
I am excited	It's a drag

Brain chemistry, food and stress

The next time someone says to you, "It's all in your mind", instead of being irritated, stop and think for a minute — in one sense this is probably correct. Our reactions to stress are governed not only by stress hormones, but also by the chemicals in our brains. The ease, or difficulty, with which our brains fire off these chemicals, is one of the key differences in how we perceive stress, how we respond to it, and what our physical reactions are.

You may be astounded to discover that the food we eat can make a radical difference to the way that these brain chemicals work. Foods can have a strong influence on specific brain chemicals called beta-endorphins, serotonin and dopamine.

BETA-ENDORPHINS

Some people have a tendency towards an increased response to brain chemicals called beta-endorphins. In extreme cases, this genetic trait can be responsible for a history of alcoholism or addictions in a family. Illicit opiate drugs, such as morphine and heroin, raise the level of beta-endorphins in the brain, and this is highly addictive.

Sugar also acts to increase beta-endorphin levels. If drugs are used to block beta-endorphin receptor sites in the brain, sugar consumption drops. Alcohol, which is a concentrated source of sugar, also affects beta-endorphins. People who have naturally low levels of beta-endorphins have a heightened response to alcohol. In other words, if the same amount of alcohol is drunk by two people, one with low beta-endorphin levels, and one with higher levels, the person with lower levels will experience a greater rise in beta-endorphins, despite having the same blood-alcohol level. This can be a significant factor in whether or not someone succumbs to addiction. Women, the overweight, and people with a family background of alcoholism or drug addiction,

are more at risk than others. Also, for women, beta-endorphin levels are lower pre-menstrually and this can increase cravings for food, sugar or chocolate during the week before a period.

SEROTONIN

Serotonin can best be described as our "satisfaction" brain chemical. When we have high levels of it, we feel good. If levels drop, we feel lousy. One of the ways of raising serotonin levels is to eat tryptophan-rich foods. Tryptophan is an amino acid (protein building block) which, amongst other functions, is converted into serotonin. Foods that contain tryptophan include meat, fish, eggs, cheese, milk, yoghurt, nuts, and legumes such as peas, beans and lentils. Turkey, cottage cheese, pheasant and partridge are particularly good sources. Eating whole carbohydrates (such as wholemeal bread, brown rice, wholewheat spaghetti and pasta, jacket potatoes and porridge oats) alongside tryptophan-rich foods, helps to force the tryptophan to go down the route of turning into serotonin. Fats and oils, sugar and alcohol do not contain tryptophan.

Alcohol, sugar and chocolate can have a powerful effect on brain chemicals. They increase levels of beta-endorphins, which make us feel good. However, they can be addictive.

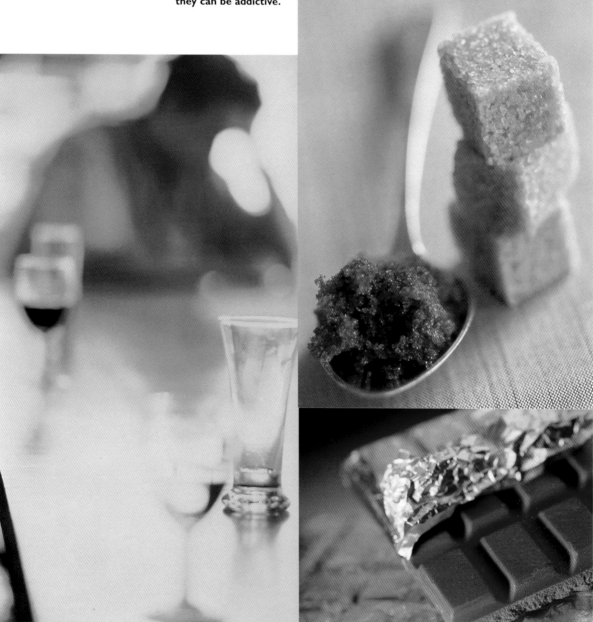

DOPAMINE

If we have low levels of dopamine, we can suffer a lack of motivation and get depressed. Some people actually prefer to be working under pressure, or occupying themselves with death-defying sporting activities. Inertia is their idea of hell – their Sundays are never spent reading the papers with their feet up. It is possible that these people are trying to replace the stimulation they would get from normal dopamine levels by revving themselves up through the use of sugar, alcohol and coffee, which provide the same stimulatory effect as stress.

Dopamine is made from tyrosine, another amino acid found in protein foods. Tyrosine is also needed for the production of adrenaline, and it has been used to help drug addicts to kick their habit by decreasing the depression, irritability and fatigue that accompanies drug withdrawal, and to help them stay off mood-enhancing drugs.

A crank is a man with a new idea – until it catches on.

MARK TWAIN

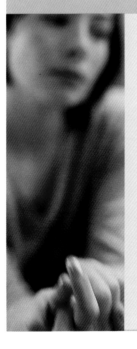

A WIN/WIN SITUATION

WIN/LOSE

We are so used to thinking in terms of winning or losing in a given situation that it can come as surprise to learn that we can always win! Everything in our society is geared up to winning or losing: sports, games, life and love; exams, job interviews or diets.

LEARN

"Losing" simply means that you have not got the result you wanted. But by changing your mind-set, you can help alter the outcome of events. Assuming that the same action always gives rise to the same outcome, changing the action will change the outcome – this is learning.

WIN/WIN

So if you view undesirable outcomes as a series of clues that will enlighten you about how to improve your technique or handling of a situation, you can create a new outcome. This means that you always win. Either you win outright, or you enhance your knowledge in such a way that you have a better chance of winning next time.

NEXT!

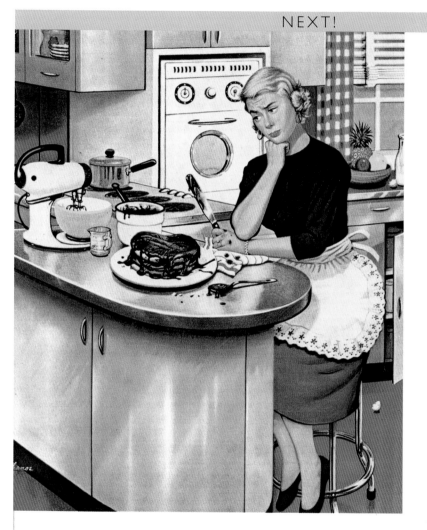

The prospect of life without chocolate may be apalling, but it's possible to find replacement indulgences.

Much stress is brought on by a sense of loss. We can't imagine being without something to which we have become accustomed, and cry, "I can't live without my ... lover/chocolate/job/wine/house/coffee" and so on. But in reality we can usually do without these things, and find new options. So if something is taken away from you, or you cut something out of your life, don't dwell on what you imagine you have lost, but think about a replacement or alternatives. There will always be another lover, or another job, and there are different things in life to enjoy instead of that fix of chocolate, wine or coffee – you just need to find what they are. I like the story that Anthony Robbins, author of *Unlimited Power*, tells of the woman who, instead of crying over her smashed love affair, goes out into the street and shouts, "Next!" There is much truth in the time-honoured sayings "Every cloud has a silver lining", "There are plenty more fish in the sea", and "There is no point crying over spilt milk".

I want it now!

As the saying goes, when the going gets tough, the tough go shopping. Why is retail therapy so satisfying? The answer is instant gratification. The same goes for our propensity for having "just one more" cream bun, piece of chocolate or beer. The diet always starts tomorrow!

The chemical rewards of instant gratification are many. For example, levels of certain brain chemicals are boosted, including serotonin, our "satisfaction" provider; the hormone adrenaline is also elevated. These processes are sparked by any addictive tendency – whether it is shopping, gambling, drinking or disordered eating.

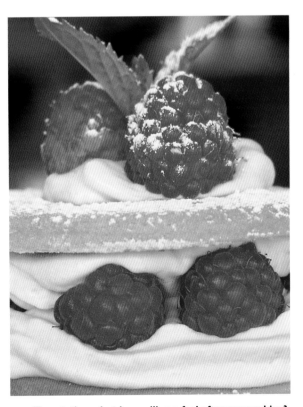

Temptation – but how will you feel after succumbing?

ENJOY NOW – PAY LATER

The principle of credit-card shopping (enjoy now and pay later) can be applied to any repeated behaviour pattern linked to instant gratification. For example, take that diet you have been meaning to start. Divide a piece of paper into two columns, "How I feel now" and "How I will feel later". Each of these is further divided into "Pros" and "Cons". Make lists of all the benefits and shortcomings of a course of action. For instance, imagine that a cream cake is sitting temptingly in front of you. Do you eat it or not?

● Answer: you eat it. You will find that your list of Pros (short-term benefits) is the driving force behind the behaviour pattern you are trying to get rid of: instant gratification. All the Cons will be long-term, meaning that you defer feeling bad in favour of feeling good now.

● Answer: you don't eat it, and choose an apple instead. Conversely, this will result in feeling bad in the short term, whilst delaying feeling good about yourself.

We are programmed to feel good *now*. This is why it is so hard to change habits.

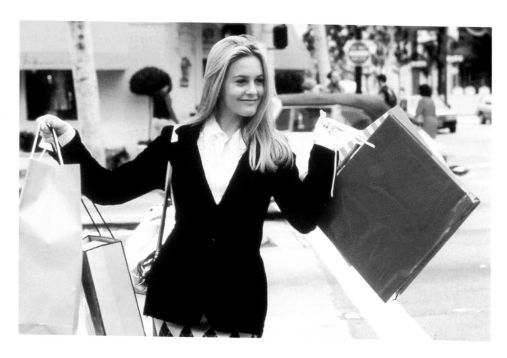

Alicia Silverstone proudly displays her haul from a round of retail therapy in *Clueless*. Addictive tendencies boost levels of serotonin, beta-endorphins and adrenaline, which is very unhelpful in the long term.

DECISION	HOW I FEEL NOW	HOW I WILL FEEL LATER
Eat cream cake	**Pros** Tastes good Gives instant energy Gives a mental boost Enjoy it Don't feel deprived Enjoy afternoon tea with friend	**Cons** Put on weight Feel bad about myself Get energy droop later Feel sick if eat too many
Eat apple instead of cream cake	**Cons** Feel hungry Feel deprived Wonder what cake tastes like Don't want to eat apple instead	**Pros** Feel virtuous Avoid blood sugar roller-coaster Not frightened of getting on scales Feel good about eating apple instead Have longer-lasting energy

Make a similar list for yourself of the pros and cons of any compulsive, addictive behaviour pattern that you have. If there are issues you need to resolve, the trick is to learn to focus on the long-term gains, enjoying and experiencing those gains now.

REPLACEMENT THERAPY

Replacement therapy means finding alternatives to activities that you want to wean yourself away from. Keep a small notebook in your bag and write down ideas as they occur to you. Remember that if they are too unrealistically virtuous, you probably won't do them: walking in the park instead of going shopping may not really work – unless you really enjoy walking in the park! Here are some initial ideas to get you started:

● Call a friend and go to a sauna together to gossip.

● Take a long bubble bath with dimmed lights, candles, some calming music and a sparkling herbal drink.

● Rent a video – a comedy will make you laugh.

● Buy a book of healthy cookery recipes and work your way through it – one recipe every time you feel like eating something unhealthy. Depending on your mood, eat it all yourself, or ask a friend round.

● Take the afternoon off to see a blockbuster movie or a theatre matinée.

● Enjoy childlike fun for a few hours – visit a museum, the funfair, or feed the ducks (borrow a child from a friend, or take your own).

● Give yourself that long-overdue pedicure or manicure.

CREATING ABUNDANCE

Have you noticed how some people are magnets for all the good things in life? They seem to sail along with a confident smile on their face, graciously enjoying all that is on offer to them. Are they just lucky, or do they have an innate ability to create abundance in their life? The answer is that these people are communicating in a way that attracts the best from other people. What they are doing, often imperceptibly, is giving something. It could be as simple as offering a smile and a pleasant greeting – which just might be enough to brighten the day of the person they are dealing with.

Giving is an art form in its own right, and the most important aspect of it is to not expect anything in return. The minute you inject selfishness into the equation, the "transaction" becomes tainted and you do not get back much at all. But if you give without expecting a return, the seeds you have sown will almost always produce a fruitful harvest. You create abundance. Experiment with this for a few weeks and see what happens. Giving pays rich dividends.

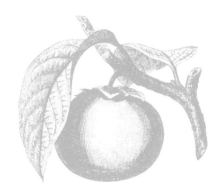

The only way to have a friend is to be one.

RALPH WALDO EMERSON

HELP OTHERS – HELP YOURSELF

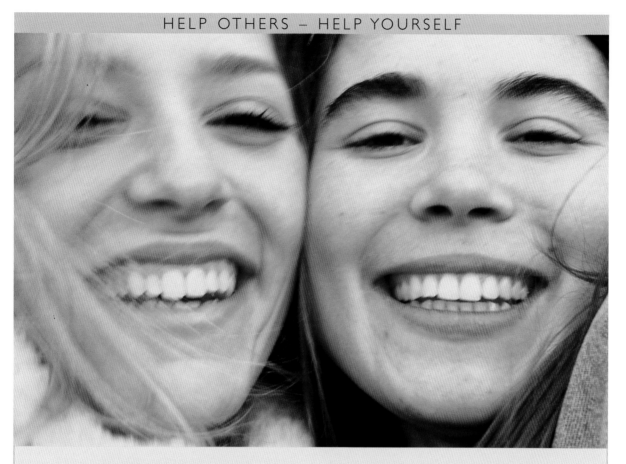

These are some things you can give:

A smile.

A greeting.

A loan of a book, or similar (not money).

Your time.

A shoulder to cry on.

Advice (but only when it is sought, and then in great moderation. It is better to listen than to talk).

Send a nice letter, e-mail or fax to someone you haven't spoken to for a while.

There are times when you should not give:

When you feel you want to say "No".

If you think you are being taken advantage of.

If you feel resentful.

When the "cost" is too high.

Can stress make you fat?

If your life is busy, and you seem to spend most of your time racing around like a headless chicken, without time to eat proper meals, this should, theoretically, ensure that you are skinny. So why do many of us put on weight when our lives are like this? Some people lose large amounts of weight when they are busy or anxious, no matter how much they eat. Others will just start to pile on the pounds, irrespective of whether or not they are eating more. If anything will compound stress, it is the wobbly spectre of weight gain!

Of course many of us do eat more when we are under stress, and comfort eating may contribute surplus calories. The quantity of food consumed may not have increased, but the composition of snacks and meals may have an increased fat and calorie content.

We tend to fall back on our favourite fixes whenever we are under stress, and these are very rarely a crunchy apple, or a soothing herbal tea. They are more likely to be sugary "energy" foods, or comfort foods such as chocolate, pasta, cheese or alcohol. Such foods commonly trigger the release of calming brain chemicals or fill the blood sugar void left after adrenaline and insulin levels have been pushed up.

INSULIN ISSUES

Stress triggers body stores to release blood sugar for instantly available energy. Blood sugar levels are also raised by eating sugary snacks, refined carbohydrates such as white bread, white rice, white pasta, and by drinking alcohol.

Insulin is a hormone designed to lower high levels of blood sugar. It brings down blood sugar levels by storing the excess in body cells: if blood sugar levels are very high, much of this sugar is converted to fat. In addition to this, the higher your blood sugar, the more insulin you release. Insulin makes you more sensitive to an enzyme called lipoprotein lipase, which makes more fat.

FAT STORAGE

Part of the stress reaction involves fat storage. Elevated levels of the stress hormone cortisol increase the storage of fat in the stomach area. This is because fat cells located deep in the abdomen seem to have more receptors for cortisol than cells at more superficial levels in the body, consequently leading to increased fat storage. The evolutionary explanation for this may be that in our cave-dwelling days, fat was physiologically coveted for its warmth and as an energy store. But our bodies do not seem to have realized that we now live in centrally-heated houses and do not have to hunt our food. The body is still saying to itself, "I'm in a crisis situation, and I need to stock up on reserves for the future, so I think I'll store a little more fat".

FOOD CRAVINGS

A short while after a crisis we can become very orally fixated. Some people are lucky and this just translates into

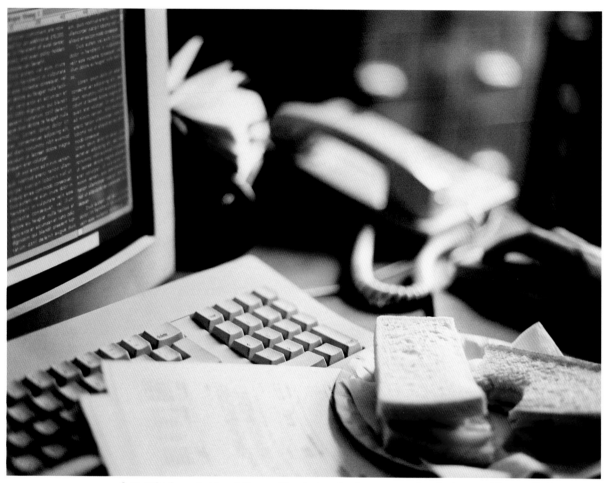

A snatched meal at lunchtime, without stopping for a proper break, does nothing to alleviate stress.

biting their fingernails. But for most people it means reverting to age-old addictions such as smoking, coffee, alcohol, sugar, chocolate, or a plate piled high with steaming pasta. If this happened on the odd occasion, then it would not matter too much. But if we are constantly in a state of anxiety, depression or fighting other stresses, it tends to happen very frequently.

Solitude permits the mind to feel.

WILLIAM WORDSWORTH

Apart from the obvious impact that these food cravings have on weight – increased fat intake and empty calories from sugar and alcohol – our favourite food fixes have another way of causing us to put on weight. Foods to which we have a sensitivity (and likely candidates include wheat, dairy products and soya), can lead to bloating, water retention and increased weight.

under **attack!**

Find out what stress can do to your body systems, and how to beat its negative effects

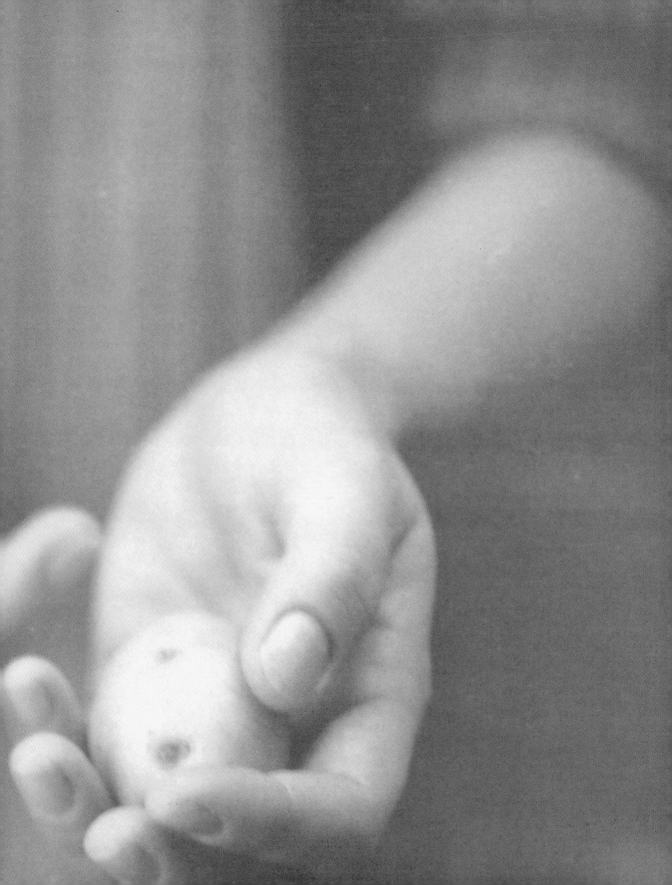

All systems go!

You are walking home down a dark road one night at the end of October. The night is still, your pace quickens, and you try to chase away thoughts of muggers lurking in every shadow. And then, your worst nightmare – out of the gloom jumps... a cat!

In that moment your physical reaction is identical to that of your forebears, the Stone Age hunter-gatherers who roamed the land looking for food and shelter. On encountering a predator, their choice was simple – fight the danger or flee from it. The body's response in such a situation is called the "fight or flight" reaction: the body meets the challenge by releasing a rush of hormones to deal with the emergency. Adrenaline, the stress hormone, has an instant effect on virtually all body systems.

The fight or flight reaction evolved as a life-saving mechanism. It is a totally appropriate reaction when, for example, you are driving a car and suddenly have to swerve to avoid an accident. It is less appropriate when the threat or stimulus is of a more mundane kind, such as a row with your partner, a tight deadline at work, or being late for an appointment. Anger, fear, frustration, excitement – all these emotions trigger an adrenaline rush to fight or flee, but our acquired cultural and social controls usually prevent us from doing either, with the result that the response remains activated for long periods and we are then not able to replenish our physical, mental or emotional reserves.

The body does not have any variations on this theme. The adrenal glands just respond to stimuli, and they are under the control of the hypothalamus in the brain. Because of this link with the brain, thoughts can, and do, act as triggers.

IN LESS THAN A SECOND, ADRENALINE WILL:

- Increase heart rate.
- Stimulate respiration.
- Relax smooth muscle in the lung bronchioles, in order to improve oxygen circulation to body tissues.
- Dilate the pupils of the eyes, to improve vision.
- Improve hearing.
- Constrict the smooth muscle of the skin, leading to gooseflesh and hair standing on end.
- Divert blood away from the process of digestion, which has the effect of slowing down digestion.
- Take blood from the skin (hence looking "pale with fear").
- Dilate arteries to improve circulation to muscles.
- Stimulate metabolism.
- Contract skeletal muscles.
- Stimulate endorphins (brain chemicals), which make pain and fatigue less noticeable.
- Mobilize liver and muscle stores of glycogen, which elevates blood sugar and supplies ready energy.
- Contract gut sphincters and urinary sphincters.
- Increase coagulability of blood to maximize repair in the event of a wound.

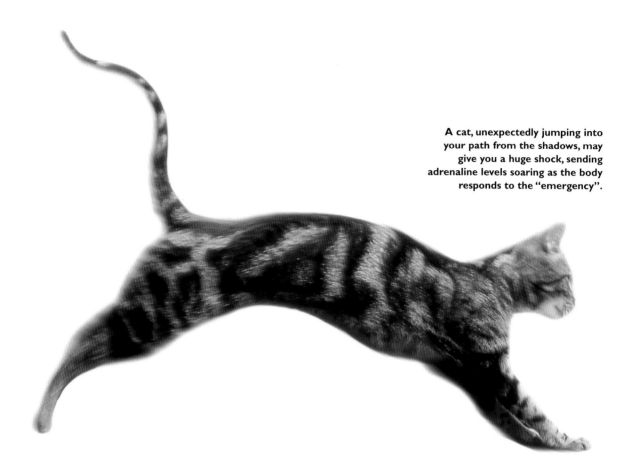

A cat, unexpectedly jumping into your path from the shadows, may give you a huge shock, sending adrenaline levels soaring as the body responds to the "emergency".

This means that if you are under any undue pressure, either physical or mental, your body will be pumping out adrenaline.

The critical thing to understand is that, because adrenaline is a survival hormone, it also takes priority over other body functions. The cost to the body of an adrenaline rush is not insignificant. It uses up large amounts of valuable nutrients –

in particular vitamins B3, B5, B6 and C, and the minerals magnesium and zinc. We will look at these in more detail later on in the book.

It is clear that excessive adrenaline production can be extremely damaging. The good news is that its negative effects can be reduced, or avoided altogether, by modulating our response and boosting our physical reserves.

Here's a two-step formula for handling stress. Step one: don't sweat the small stuff; step two: remember, it's all small stuff.

ANTHONY ROBBINS

Stress and your hormone system

The adrenal glands are tiny organs that sit on top of each kidney. Their health is paramount to our general health, because in addition to producing the hormone adrenaline, which has such powerful effects on the whole body, they produce other hormones.

The body's hormone system is highly interconnected, with each hormone affecting others in a complex feedback system. It is rather like a performance by an orchestra: if one section of the orchestra is out of harmony, the music being played sounds terrible. Hormones also need to be in tune, or the body's overall balance is upset. The stress hormones adrenaline, noradrenaline and cortisol have a direct impact on other hormone systems, chiefly blood sugar regulation, sex hormones and thyroid hormones.

The inner part of the adrenal gland, the medulla, produces adrenaline and noradrenaline, which are concerned with the immediate reactions to stress in the fight or flight response. The outer part of the adrenal gland, the cortex, is involved in dealing with longer term stress, such as illness or injury. The hormones produced in the cortex also help to regulate glucose metabolism, water balance, acid–alkaline balance and sex hormone balance.

OTHER ADRENAL HORMONES

Noradrenaline is the sister hormone to adrenaline, and together they create the fight or flight response, though they have different effects and responsibilities. The mineralocorticoids, also produced by the adrenal glands, are responsible for water and mineral balance in the body.

Cortisol is normally secreted in a rhythm over the course of 24 hours. Levels are raised in the daytime, when we are active and need its energy-boosting properties, and lower at night, when the body repairs tissues. Problems arise when we are under a lot of stress, causing our levels of cortisol to remain raised at night. When this happens, we do not feel rested after a night's sleep, and our body tissues do not repair themselves as efficiently as they might do.

A high level of cortisol also tips DHEA out of balance. DHEA is termed the "youth" hormone and is needed to keep us in prime health. If DHEA is suppressed, it can contribute to chronic fatigue syndrome as well as to early ageing.

BLOOD SUGAR

One of the main effects of raised adrenaline is that it triggers an increase in the hormone glucagon. Glucagon is responsible for releasing stored glucose, in the form of glycogen, from our muscles and liver. It is designed to give an immediate boost of energy in the event of an emergency. This is how people acquire an amazing surge of energy when faced with a life-threatening situation – for example a

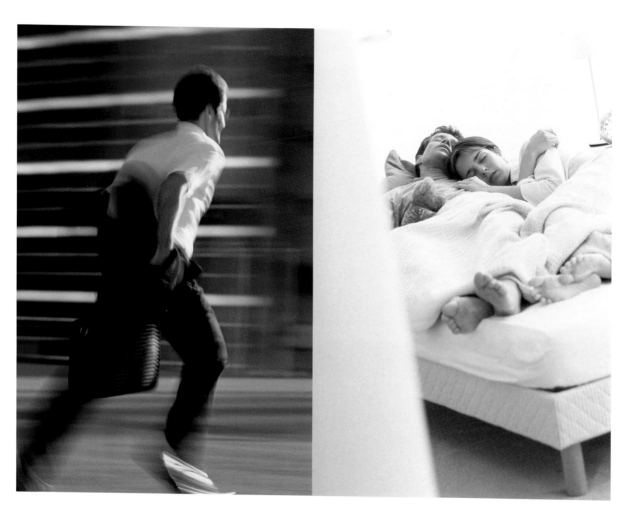

mother, who has never run in her life, sprinting to save her child from danger, in a time that would set world records.

Other factors that push up blood sugar levels are sugar in the diet, refined starches (such as white bread), caffeine and alcohol. The body does not like constantly elevated blood sugar – it leads to diabetes – so insulin is brought into play to bring blood sugar down. When this happens too often, the whole system becomes trigger-happy, and blood sugar is brought down too quickly, too often, and to too low a level. This roller-coaster effect leads to increased cravings for

Raised adrenaline triggers the release of glycogen, immediately boosting blood sugar and energy. But when blood sugar is continually fluctuating because of adrenaline, it causes symptoms such as sleepiness during the day.

anything to boost blood sugar again, and for the adrenaline rush. Symptoms that can be felt when blood sugar is fluctuating wildly include low energy levels, mood swings, insomnia, anxiety, tension, the need to sleep during the day, depression, cravings for sweet foods and addictions.

SEX HORMONES

Sex hormones are also linked to blood sugar balance. Many women notice this effect in the week before a period, when the sex hormones oestrogen and progesterone are at a high level. Cravings for sugar, chocolate or carbohydrates are often experienced at this time, together with an increased need for stimulants and "props".

The sex hormones are principally released from the ovaries or the testes, but a significant amount are released from the adrenal glands (around 25 per cent). This means that if the adrenal glands are producing an excessive adrenaline and cortisol output (or are exhausted), sex hormones will also be affected. In fact, disturbed body chemistry affects them both even more intimately – they are both made from the same substance, cholesterol.

Sex hormones are closely linked to adrenaline and noradrenaline, which are released into the bloodstream during and after sex. Sexual climax is one of the most potent – though transitory – health and mood boosters known. This may also be why, along with other "fixes", it is possible to become a "sex addict" – although it is perhaps wise to retain a degree of scepticism for those claiming it! The other side of the coin is that one in five people blames stress for diminished libido or loss of pleasure in lovemaking.

Burt Lancaster and Deborah Kerr find out that sex is one of the most potent mood boosters.

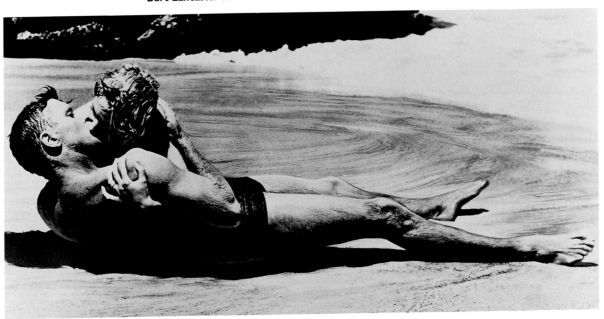

Think of solutions, not problems.

ANON

THYROID HORMONES

The thyroid gland governs our metabolism, and thyroid hormones are also affected by stress. It is quite common for an overfunctioning or underfunctioning thyroid gland to be exacerbated by too much stress. Symptoms that may suggest disturbed thyroid function include:

Overactive thyroid

Elevated body temperature
"Bulging" eyes
A tendency to be underweight
A tendency to be hyperactive

Underactive thyroid

Excessive tiredness
A tendency to put on weight
Sensitivity to cold
Blood sugar regulation problems
Low blood pressure

RELAXATION EXERCISE

■ Set a timer to go off in 5, 10 or 15 minutes' time. Lie or sit in a comfortable position. Ensure that you are warm and loosen any tight clothing.

■ Relax the larger muscles in your shoulders and neck, along with all the tiny muscles in your forehead, cheeks, jaw, around your eyes, behind your ears, chin, and even in your scalp. By concentrating on your facial muscles, the muscles in the rest of your body will also relax.

■ When your face is totally relaxed, start listening to the sounds in the room. Then listen to the sounds that are further away from your immediate surroundings – on another floor, in the street, in a nearby park. When the timer goes off, become aware of yourself in the room again, stretch, yawn if you want to, and get up. You will feel refreshed and have renewed energy.

HOMEOPATHIC REMEDIES

Homeopathic remedies may help to reduce stress. Mild formulations are available from pharmacists and healthfood shops. If you feel that you need stronger or personally tailored remedies, consult a qualified homeopath or a homeopathic doctor. The following remedies may be useful:

Tiger lily

■ *Bryonia alba* (wild hop). For anger, peevishness and irritability.
■ *Lilium tigrinum* (tiger lily). For quick-changing moods, anger, listlessness and despair.
■ *Belladonna* (deadly nightshade). For restlessness, poor sleep and tearfulness.
■ *Nux vomica* (poison nut). For irritability and early-morning waking.
■ *Ignatia amara* (St. Ignatius' bean). For severe grief accompanied by sighing and oversensitivity to pain.
■ *Pulsatilla* (anemone). For acute fear.

Stress and immune health

We have all noticed that when we are under pressure, perhaps doing too much and burning the candle at both ends, we are more vulnerable to catching any bugs that are currently doing the rounds. The body's immune system is like a defence army. In response to a threat, it produces one million white blood cells in one minute. These white blood cells are like soldiers who patrol our blood and lymph systems to seek out invaders. This is what happens when a bug launches an assault. After identifying the enemy, the soldiers call in reinforcements from other white blood cells to attack and overcome it. Finally, they dispose of the debris.

Signs that this battle between immune system and invader is going on include reddening, inflammation, mucus, pus, swollen glands and a raised temperature. The enemies may be viruses, bacteria, undigested food particles, yeasts, allergens such as pollen, body cells that have mutated (as in cancer), or parasites. Dealing with all these threats is a big job. The digestive tract plays an important part too, because it is one of the chief barriers between our inside world and the outside world. Any foods that have not been properly digested are quick to be identified, at this front line, as enemies from the outside world.

Raised stress levels have been shown to lower the white blood cell count and this can leave us open to any number of invaders. Numbers of NK cells (natural killer cells – a type of white blood cell that is one of our most important defences against cancer) are reduced by stress. Other immune problems are made much worse by stress. For instance, more fatal asthma attacks are suffered by children who are under severe stress.

Why, at a time when we need our immune system to be working at peak efficiency, precisely because we are stressed, does it fail us? Nutrition is a significant factor – both the immune system and the stress response system are heavy users of the same nutrients. So if we are experiencing high levels of stress, a call is being made on the very reserves we need to fight an immune system threat efficiently. Consequently the invading virus, bacteria, yeast, or parasite gets the upper hand, condemning us to a long drawn-out battle in order to beat it and regain our health. The nutrients that both the stress and immune systems need in large quantities are vitamins A, B, C and E, zinc, magnesium, selenium, and essential fatty acids.

He who laughs, lasts.

ANON

TOP FIVE IMMUNE SYSTEM BOOSTERS

1 Vitamin A is highly protective of mucous membranes. If the mucous membranes of the nasal and breathing passages are working properly, viruses have less chance of getting across this "barrier".

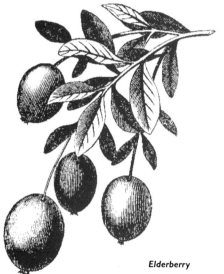

Elderberry

2 Elderberry cordial (or any drink made from a dark red fruit) is rich in proanthocyanins, which are powerhouses of support for the immune system.

3 Echinacea root capsules and tinctures have been shown to increase the activity of white blood cells.

4 Garlic stimulates the number of immune cells, and is antibacterial, antiviral and antiparasitic.

Ginger is warming and improves circulation. It also has an antiseptic effect on the lungs, making it helpful for treating colds and flu.

5 Digestive health is paramount for the health of the immune system. If you think you are allergic or sensitive to any foods, cut them out, because they will suppress your immune system.

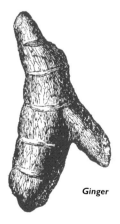

Ginger

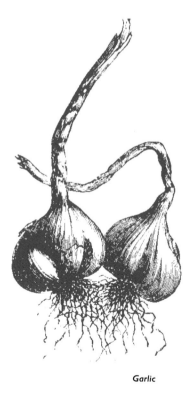

Garlic

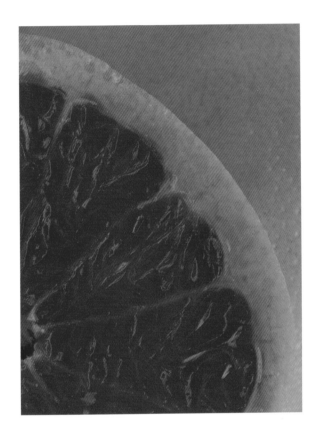

DRINKS TO STIMULATE THE IMMUNE SYSTEM

A LARGE GLASS of freshly squeezed orange and grapefruit juice provides 250mg of vitamin C. For an extra boost, add some vitamin C powder.

MAKE A SOUP from shiitake mushrooms (dried or fresh), onions, fresh crushed garlic and miso. All have proven stimulatory actions. Instead of a soup, by using less water you can make a savoury sauce that can be served with brown rice.

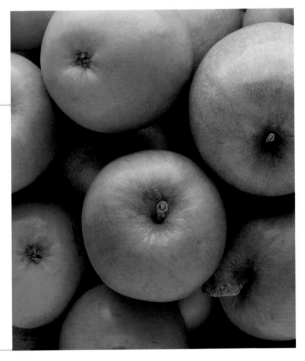

APPLE TEA is pleasantly cooling if you have a high temperature, but it can be enjoyed at any time. Wash, core and slice two cooking apples, leaving the peel on. Put them in a heatproof jar with 750ml (24fl.oz /3 cups) of filtered water. Stand the jar in a pan of water, and simmer for two hours. Remove the liquid in the jar and strain it. Add a teaspoonful of fresh lemon juice and a teaspoonful of honey. Drink warm or cold.

CAT'S CLAW is a herb, available in tea bags, that helps to increase the defences of the immune system against viruses, bacteria and even pollen (so can be useful against hay fever).

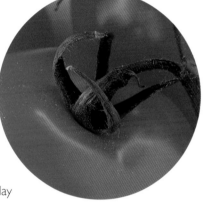

TOMATO JUICE is loaded with the antioxidant lycopene, which may be protective against certain cancers. Once a day you can also add in a 200mcg drop of the mineral selenium (sold in liquid form) along with a dash of tabasco and celery salt. Selenium is needed for the antioxidant glutathione peroxidase enzyme we manufacture in our bodies.

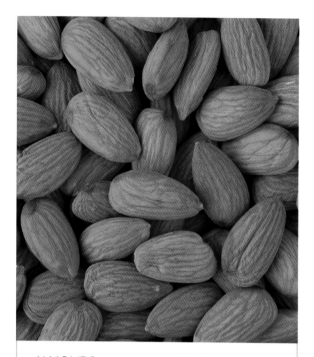

ALMONDS are recommended when you have a cold or fever. Crush 25g (1oz/¼ cup) of organic almonds in a food processor. Slowly add in up to four tablespoons of filtered water until a paste is formed. Stir in one teaspoonful of honey, then add sufficient boiling water to make a drink. Let it cool, then whizz up in the blender until frothy.

LIVE YOGHURT is a strong stimulator of the immune system. Try making a delicious yoghurt "shake", blending in lots of dark red berries for their potent antioxidant qualities.

JAPANESE GREEN TEA is an immune system stimulant, which has been extensively studied. Drink it ten times a day to derive maximum benefit from the tannins, antioxidants, polyphenols and epigallocatechin gallate (the main active compound) it contains. You can buy green tea combined with other herbs such as mint.

Stress and your digestive system

The stress reaction closes down our digestive system, shunting blood away from the digestive tract towards the skeletal muscles to prepare for fight or flight. The modern result of constant, chronic stress is interrupted and disturbed digestion.

The fight or flight response, resulting from stress, diverts blood away from the digestive system. Chronic stress, therefore, puts a strain on the digestive system and causes problems.

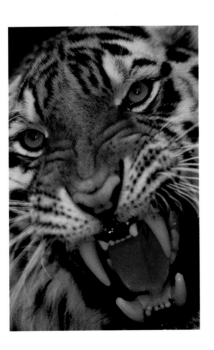

TWO BRAINS

It is now being suggested that as well as a brain in the skull, we have a type of brain in the gut. They are interconnected, so when one is upset, the other is as well. Nearly every substance that controls the brain has also been found in the gut, including all the chemical messengers such as serotonin, dopamine, glutamine and noradrenaline. The gut also contains about 24 neurochemicals, including enkephalins, which have an opiate-like effect, and benzodiazepines, a family of psychoactive chemicals that includes popular drugs such as the tranquillizer, Valium.

DIGESTIVE DISEASES

Digestive complaints such as irritable bowel syndrome (IBS) and stomach ulcers are linked to dietary imbalances, especially to a lack of foods containing fibre. However, only a certain number of people recover when their diet is addressed – for a very large proportion of people, stress is the basis of their digestive complaints.

When under stress (usually a long period of emotional stress), the impact on the digestive tract is great. The effect of blood being directed away from the digestive tract means that the squeezing motion (peristalsis) that moves food along the tract is inhibited. This can either cause it to go into spasm, or to be flaccid, contributing to the intermittent bouts of diarrhoea and constipation known as IBS. Stress may

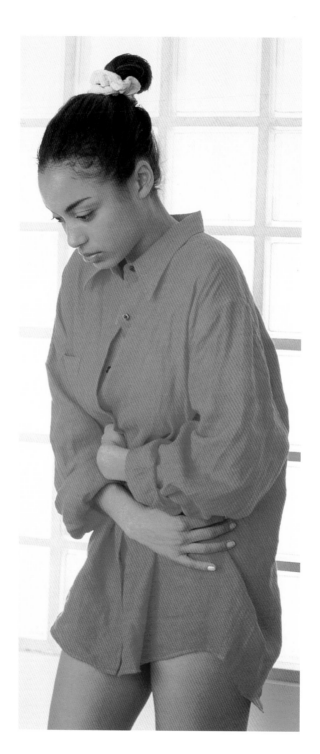

Irritable bowel syndrome is a stress-related disease, causing bouts of diarrhoea and constipation. Stomach ulcers are also induced by stress.

lower or step up the production of stomach acid, both of which can cause stomach ulcers. If stomach acid is increased, and the mucous membrane lining the digestive tract damaged, the acid can literally burn a hole in the stomach or duodenal tissues. If stomach acid is decreased, the organism *Helicobacter pylori* may survive in the body, which eats away the same tissues. If the stress hormone, cortisol, is constantly elevated at times when it is meant to be low, this will impair healing of the tissues of the gut wall.

LEAKY GUT

As has already been discussed, cortisol levels are intended to be low at night, which is when we rest and when body tissues are repaired. But if we are in a state of constant stimulation, or sleep is interrupted regularly, or if we take stimulants that trigger cortisol, then this repair cannot, and does not, take place efficiently.

If the gut is not repaired regularly, it can become permeable, or leaky, a little like a colander. It begins to let microscopic, partially digested food particles into the bloodstream. This increased permeability, exacerbated by stress and other factors, increases the chance of an allergic reaction to everyday foods in the diet, and this can result in a number of seemingly unconnected symptoms. These include bloating, indigestion, flatulence, constipation, loose stools, diarrhoea, headaches, migraines, eczema, psoriasis and urticaria. It may not be obvious that the symptoms are linked to food sensitivity and to gut leakiness, because they often occur several hours, or even the next day, after eating the problem foods.

This condition can also be triggered by the fact that when we are stressed, we tend to increase our intake of certain substances. For instance, we use sugar and refined carbohydrates to fuel our blood sugar swings, we depend on alcohol to calm our nerves or to help us relax, and we swallow painkillers to ease headaches and other pains. All these things directly, or indirectly, contribute to making the digestive tract more porous.

STOP THE VICIOUS CYCLE

There are a number of things that can be done to improve digestive function by toning the gut and helping to heal it. The first objective is to eliminate those factors that might be triggering the permeability. The next step is to introduce substances that will help to heal the gut wall.

FACTORS THAT CAUSE GUT PERMEABILITY

- Stress
- Sugar
- Refined carbohydrates (such as white bread, white rice, white pasta, most pastry, peeled potatoes and potato products).
- High alcohol intake.
- Aspirin and other non-steroidal painkillers or anti-inflammatories.
- Food sensitivities (most commonly wheat or dairy).
- Insufficient fibre in the diet.

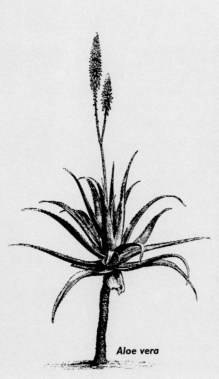

Aloe vera

TO SOOTHE A LEAKY GUT

- Aloe vera juice, diluted with water.
- Slippery elm (tea or supplements).
- Marshmallow (capsules or powder).
- Liquorice (deglycyrrhized).
- Oatbran oil or rice bran oil.
- Psyllium husks – build up slowly to two teaspoons twice a day.

DIGESTIVE AIDS

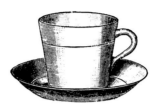

GINGER TEA Familiar as an anti-nausea remedy. It is powerful against all types of digestive disquiet, including morning sickness and travel sickness.

MINT TEA Mint and peppermint have a long history of use for stomach problems. Drinking several cups a day is one of the most powerful stomach settlers known.

CARROT JUICE A rich source of beta-carotene, which converts to vitamin A and helps to heal mucous membranes in the gut.

CABBAGE JUICE Contains high levels of a substance called glutamine, which is a powerful repairer of the gut wall and helps to maintain healthy mucous membranes. Because cabbage juice is strong-tasting, drink it in a mixture with other juices, one part cabbage juice to three parts carrot (or other) juice.

GROUND SEEDS Increase your levels of zinc and essential fatty acids, both of which help to repair damage to the digestive tract. Ground seeds such as sunflower, pumpkin, sesame, linseed and hemp can be sprinkled into a juice drink.

The secret of success is making your vocation your vacation.

MARK TWAIN

Stress and cardiovascular health

The cardiovascular system consists of a pump, the heart, and several miles of arteries and veins which eventually subdivide into the microscopic capillaries that link to every single cell in the body. These capillaries carry blood, which supplies proteins and fats to the cells, glucose and oxygen for energy, and takes away waste products and carbon dioxide. It also circulates the white cells of the immune system to guard against any troublemakers. Every cell in the body is dependent upon a correctly functioning cardiovascular system.

Constant arguments, as demonstrated here by Richard Burton and Elizabeth Taylor, push blood pressure up.

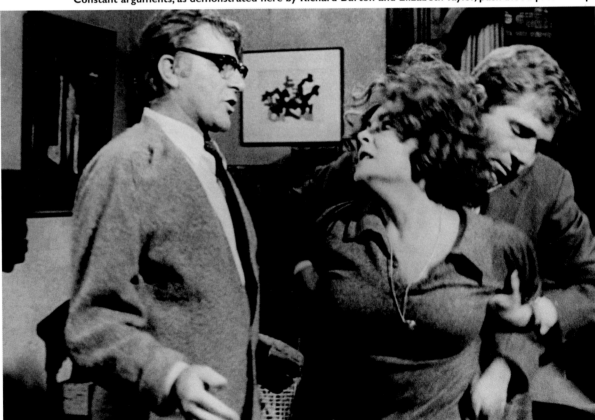

Signs that something may be going wrong include high blood pressure, raised cholesterol levels (especially "bad" LDL cholesterol), blocked arteries, angina, and eventually thrombosis, a heart attack or a stroke. Heart disease has been called the silent time-bomb because it takes many years for noticeable symptoms to reveal themselves, and by then a lot of damage has already taken place. Acute stress definitely puts the cardiovascular system into crisis – when people are bereaved, their risk of a heart attack within the following 24 hours increases 14 times.

Women are frequently complacent about cardiovascular disease because it is mistakenly thought to be a man's disease. While women are menstruating they are protected by their hormones to a degree, but after the menopause the risk for women is identical to that of men.

ARGUE YOUR WAY TO A HEART ATTACK

One of the main contributors to cardiovascular disease is chronic stress. Arguments, anxiety, tension and repressed emotions all raise adrenaline levels, which by contracting and hardening the arteries over time, raises blood pressure. The short-term effects of stress hormones can be felt as an increased pulse rate, pounding heart and perhaps a pulsing of the veins at the side of the head. If stress continues for a long time, then long-term damage to the structure of the cardiovascular system may result.

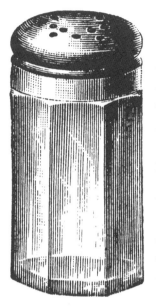

EAT YOUR WAY TO A HEART ATTACK

Salt is a villain. It raises blood pressure by increasing fluid retention in the arteries. The combination of stress and a high-salt diet can have a devastating effect on a person's risk of heart disease.

When we are under a lot of stress, or are anxious or depressed, we often turn to our favourite "props", such as alcohol, coffee and tea; sometimes we use over-the-counter medicines to alleviate muscular tension or headaches. These substances need to be processed and disarmed by the liver. The liver is critical to the health of the cardiovascular system because it is where cholesterol is made and processed by the body. Raised cholesterol levels imply that the liver is not doing its job properly, perhaps because it is overloaded by having to process all the substances we tend to take when under increased pressure. Many other factors are also involved in heart disease, including genetic predisposition, lack of exercise, smoking, saturated fat intake and body weight.

Don't refuse to go on an occasional wild goose chase.

That's what wild geese are for.

ANON

Stress and your nervous system

When we are under stress for any period of time, the brain is affected. Our minds seem woolly, concentration wavers, moods are affected and sleeping rhythm destroyed. In the worst cases, it can lead to depression and mental health problems. It is common to hear people attribute their stress to "nerves", and they are right to do so. Stress first affects the parts of the body that are related to the nervous system: signs include irritability, high blood pressure, headaches, dizziness, neckaches, loss of appetite, and stress-related digestive symptoms.

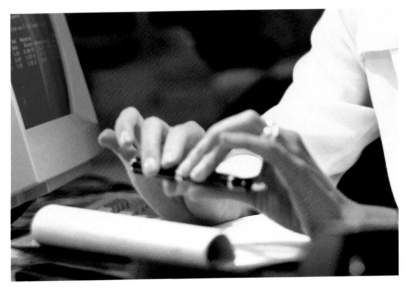

When you pick up a pen, the nerves that perform the task are under your conscious control. But nervous system functions that work of their own accord, such as the heart, are very vulnerable to stress hormones.

The nervous system is divided into two sections: voluntary and autonomic. The voluntary nervous system is conscious and each time you pick up a pen, scratch your nose or do the tango, you are bringing this system into play. The autonomic nervous system, on the other hand, is under less conscious control. This system is linked to organs such as the heart, lungs and kidneys, which work without us being aware of them. It also triggers blushing, goosebumps, sweating and sexual arousal. The autonomic nervous system is affected by adrenaline.

The autonomic system is further divided into the sympathetic and parasympathetic branches. These have opposing effects to each other – one will speed up heart rate, while the other slows it down. One will divert blood to the muscles, while the other reverses the process. One will cause you to shiver, while the other stops it. Stress hormones work on the sympathetic system, at the expense of the parasympathetic system, and cause heightened nervous stimulation for long periods of time. This is rather like keeping your foot on the body's accelerator pedal all the time, wearing down your health and causing exhaustion.

REFLEXOLOGY RELAXATION SESSION

Reflexology has a positive effect on the whole body. Get together with a friend and arrange to work on each other's feet once a week. Complete the exercise on one foot before moving on to the other foot. By relaxing both feet, tensions will drift away.

1. FREE UP THE FOOT AND ANKLE

Cradling the heel with one hand, use the other hand to gently but firmly circle the foot at the ankle joint. Then take the foot between both hands and carefully, but rapidly, rock it from side to side.

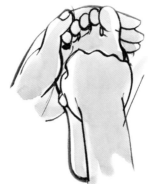

2. KNEADING THE SOLE OF THE FOOT

Push your fist (either one) into the sole of the foot, with the opposite hand over the top of the foot. Press your fist into the sole as if you are kneading dough, while exerting an opposite pressure with your other hand. Start off slowly and set up a gentle rhythm.

3. USING PRESSURE POINTS TO RELAX BREATHING

Press your thumbs into the sole of the foot and work all your fingers, on either side, towards the middle of the foot. Then, with your thumbs, work the sole of the foot from the "diaphragm" line (see far right) to the base of each toe. Finally, work the top of the foot. Use your thumbs to massage from the junctions between the toes along the grooves made by the metatarsals.

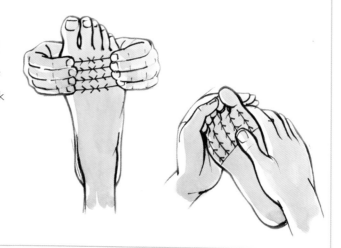

TOP FIVE MIND CALMERS

1 Ylang-ylang essential oil pacifies the mind, dispels anger and stubbornness while creating a feeling of peace. It also enhances sensuality. Add a few drops to your bath.

2 Oats have a calming effect. Try porridge, oatcakes, oat flapjacks and oats flaked into soups and casseroles.

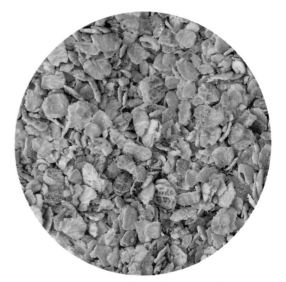

3 St. John's wort (hypericum) is a natural antidepressant, which allows the brain to process pleasurable feelings instead of blocking them. It does this by restoring the communication links between nerve endings, helping to lift low moods, and banish despair and anxiety.

Oats and chamomile soothe mental stress.

4 Herbal infusions with calming effects include chamomile, lime flower, skullcap and hawthorn. Buy herbs from a reputable herbalist to ensure quality. Leave to steep for at least 15 minutes before drinking.

5 Meditation is an effective way of encouraging alpha and theta brain waves, which are typical of the state of deep relaxation.

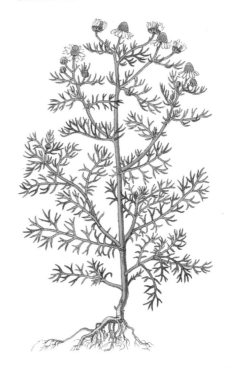

ESSENTIAL OILS

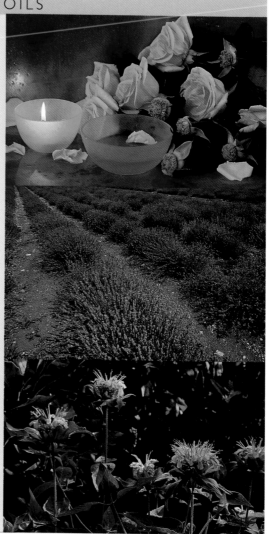

The olfactory lobe in the brain, which interprets smell, is connected to the emotional, or limbic, brain. The limbic brain plays a cental role in the senses of pain, pleasure, happiness, sadness, joy, anger, fear, sexual arousal, memory and interpretation of experiences. The connection between the two is the reason why the essential oils of plants can directly affect our moods and emotions. If you are pregnant, essential oils must only be used with professional advice from an qualified aromatherapist. Add four to six drops of essential oils to a warm bath, or dilute them in a base oil such as almond oil and dab behind the ears.

For fatigue: rosemary, lemon, lemongrass, eucalyptus, peppermint, jasmine.

For anxiety: lavender, marjoram, bergamot, basil, neroli, ylang-ylang, juniper.

For loneliness and heartbreak: rose oil (the ultimate woman's oil for comfort and self-indulgence – expensive, but can be bought more economically in scented room sprays).

For anxiety and depression: bergamot with basil and clary sage.

For nervous tension: bergamot with lavender, neroli with marjoram, lavender with juniper, ylang-ylang and basil.

For insomnia: bergamot, lavender, marjoram, ylang-ylang, juniper, basil, clary sage.

You must begin to trust yourself.
If you do not, then you will forever be looking to others to prove
your own merit to you, and you will never be satisfied.

JANE ROBERTS

Stress and your framework

As we have already seen, the physical effects of stress hormones are widespread. One of their main effects is to contract skeletal muscles. The contraction of these muscles may be quite subtle, so it is not immediately noticeable. However, if one muscle (or set of muscles) is contracted, then another opposing muscle (or set of muscles) must be elongated. It is a bit like the guy ropes on the mast of a boat. If one rope is overtight, the opposite rope will be longer, and the mast will tilt slightly. Alterations in how we hold our skeleton can, over time, lead to the body compensating so that, for instance, tension in the shoulders may affect the hips. Interrelated tensions may give rise to long-term chronic neck and back strain, or pain in other areas.

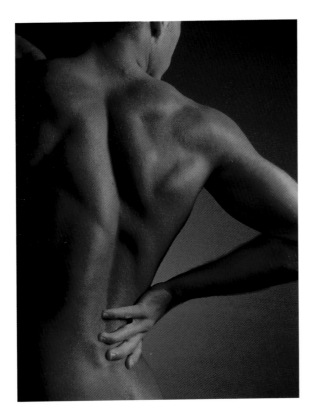

Back problems affect many people, and are often due to the tensing of muscles over a long period.

Muscles that are permanently (although subtly) tense are much more susceptible to injuries such as strains, sprains and torn muscles. If tensions go on for too long, or are repeatedly aggravated, then the joints will eventually suffer wear and tear and osteoarthritis can set in.

To make matters worse, raised levels of cortisol suppress levels of human growth hormone, and limit the ability of the tissues to heal themselves. One study found that the length of time it took for wounds to heal was an average of nine days longer in people who scored high in psychological stress tests.

SKIN, HAIR AND NAILS

Our skin is an outer reflection of our inner health. Hair and nails are a further extension of this – they are dead tissue, but reflect the state of our health at the time they are growing. The skin, hair and nails are intimately affected by stress. Anybody who breaks out in a rash or has an eczema attack when under pressure will be aware of this. Prematurely greying hair may be a sign of selenium deficiency, because selenium is used up in huge volumes by one of the main liver detoxification enzymes, glutathione peroxidase. Hair that turns grey or thins earlier than expected is often attributed to high levels of stress. A Chinese saying sums up the effects of stress on hair well: "Grass doesn't grow well on a busy street".

Nutrients needed for skin, hair and nail repair include vitamin C, for collagen building, B-vitamins, for strong hair and nails, and zinc, which is used for protein (and therefore skin, nail and hair) manufacture. However, the stress reaction uses up huge quantities of these important nutrients.

TOP FIVE SKIN SMOOTHERS

1 Drink two litres (3½pts/10 cups) of filtered or mineral water a day. Water helps our detoxification systems and is a valuable source of calcium. The skin is our largest organ of elimination and is cleared by hydration and detoxification.

2 Eat five portions of fruit a day. Fruits such as blackberries, cherries, strawberries and loganberries, are rich sources of proanthocyanins, which protect against skin destruction and wrinkles. Fruit is also rich in vitamin C, which builds collagen.

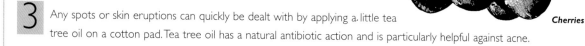

Cherries

3 Any spots or skin eruptions can quickly be dealt with by applying a little tea tree oil on a cotton pad. Tea tree oil has a natural antibiotic action and is particularly helpful against acne.

4 One of the greatest favours you can do for your skin is to break open a capsule of vitamin E oil and spread it over your skin a couple of times a week. The oil is absorbed quickly and it helps to make baby-soft skin. You can also rub it on a wound to improve healing and reduce scarring.

5 Use cabbage as a skin healer. Put fresh dark green cabbage leaves in the fridge to chill, crush them to slightly bruise them and then apply them to any inflamed area of skin. The live enzymes in the cabbage leaves will help to soothe the area and break down dead cells on the surface. Mashed papaya is also a treat for the skin.

Before enlightenment: chopping wood, carrying water.

After enlightenment: chopping wood, carrying water.

ZEN PROVERB

CHAPTER THREE

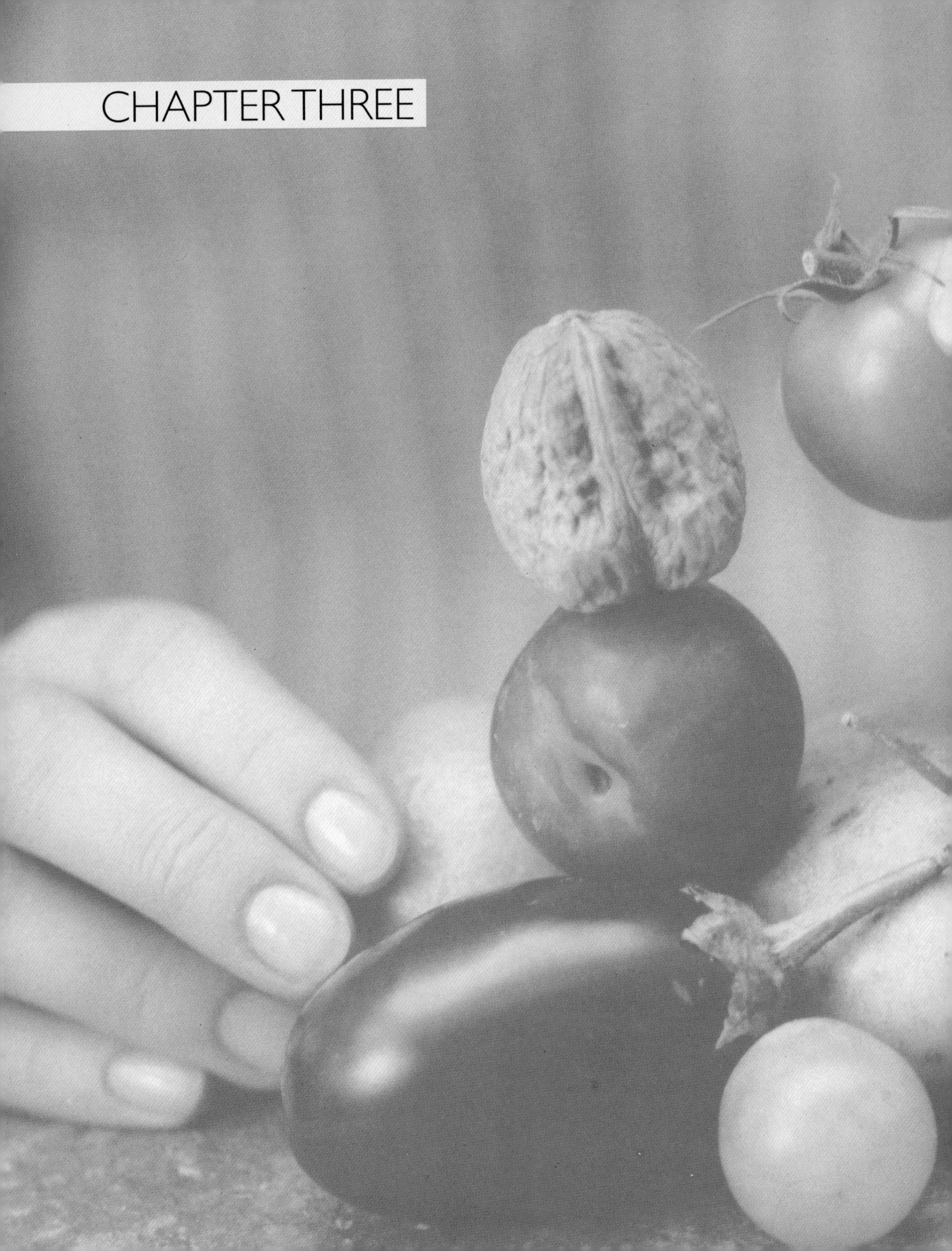

the architect
within us

How to tackle stress through diet, balance moods, increase energy and boost vitality

Food for mind and body

Food is utilized by the body for building cells. The quality of our food is vital in order to ensure that the body repairs itself properly. The lining of the gut takes around four days to renew itself; tissues in the long bones of the thigh take two to four years. So every mouthful of food you swallow determines the health of your cells and organs, and their ability to function.

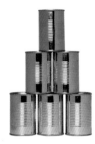

Food also provides the building blocks for the body's "messengers", chemical compounds such as nerve chemicals (neurochemicals), hormones and enzymes, which enable it to operate effectively. Every beat of your heart, every thought, and every breath you take are all governed by these messengers. If they do not work properly, your body does not work properly.

Finally, the foods we eat also have a pharmacological effect. This can be as strong as that of the medicines you may be tempted to take from time to time. While foods take longer to achieve a healing effect, they do not have the same side-effects as medicines.

THE MIND–BODY LINK

This is the medical equivalent of the chicken and egg question. Where do you start to treat someone with a physical problem – with the mind? Where do you start to treat someone with a mental problem – with the physical body? The answer is to do both. If you have a torn muscle, by all means bind it up and do gentle physiotherapy exercises, but also work on relaxation and meditation techniques to speed up healing. If you are depressed, you can certainly go for counselling, but you should also look to see whether any

vitamins and minerals are lacking in your diet, or whether you are taking in too many stimulants – both factors which adversely affect brain function. This holistic approach (treating the whole person) is not always taken by conventional physicians, but it is a "missing link" that you are quite able to address for yourself.

In Eastern medicine, the intimate link between mind and body has always been considered to impact on health. In Western medicine, stress was the first "phenomenon" to suggest that mind and body play a part in disease and the maintenance of health. The action of the adrenal glands reveals this. They are involved in a complex feedback operation with the pituitary and hypothalamus glands, known as the HPA (hypothalamus, pituitary, adrenal) axis. The hypothalamus is not only an endocrine gland secreting hormones, but is also a part of the brain. A simple thought, such as visualizing a meeting with the bank manager to discuss an overdraft, can trigger a series of physical symptoms via the HPA feedback mechanism: a pounding heart, sweating, and a churning stomach. This shows the direct effect of the mind upon the body. However, the reverse is also true – not only does the management of mental stress have a profound and positive effect on physical health, but foods have a remarkable ability to balance moods, promote healing, and increase energy and vitality.

THE KEY ELEMENTS OF YOUR DIET

The body is able to synthesize an astounding array of nutrients. However, there are around 44 to 47 nutrients that are essential to our well-being and survival, which we can only get from the diet, because the body is incapable of manufacturing them. The essential nutrients consist of 13 vitamins, 21 to 22 minerals, eight to 10 amino acids (protein building blocks), and two essential fatty acids. Our requirement for all these nutrients is one of the strongest arguments for a varied diet, as no one food, or food group, can supply everything. If our diet lacks any nutrients, it is yet another stress on the body. The science of nutrition is heading into a new era. The wisdom of thousands of years of herbalism, phytotherapy and dietary manipulation is now being substantiated by a wide body of research studying the active compounds in foods. These compounds account for what was previously viewed as seemingly magical properties. Vitamins and minerals were only identified in the last century, and scientists continue to discover more about their far-reaching implications for health. Phytonutrients, such as lycopene, quercitin and anthocyanins, are not considered essential in the conventional sense – in other words there are no deficiency diseases attributed to a lack of them. However, they are recognized to be critical for optimum health, because their strong antioxidant properties help to protect us from a wide range of diseases. Enzymes undoubtedly have a major impact on our health. They help to break down

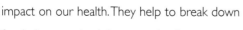

food, clean up dead tissues, and enhance our own enzyme capacity. Enzymes are destroyed by processing and cooking. By eating a wide range of foods, as close to their original state as possible, our bodies can enjoy all these benefits. But if we eat a high proportion of processed foods, we lose out on vital ingredients.

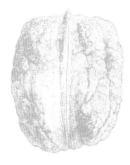

In the next few sections, we will look at the key elements of our diet, and how they relate to stress. This knowledge builds towards the Stress Protection Plan.

Carbohydrate cravings

Carbohydrates are made from carbon, hydrogen and oxygen by plants and this group of nutrients include sugars, starches and fibres of different sorts. Carbohydrates are key players in the Stress Protection Plan. They are our main source of energy, and are found in grains, pulses, fruit, vegetables, sugar and alcohol. But to support your body against the ravages of stress, it is important to consider the type, quantity and balance of carbohydrates you consume. If you choose the right kinds of carbohydrate, they will sustain you through thick and thin. If you choose the wrong type, you run the risk of sabotaging your energy levels, triggering unhelpful brain chemicals and encouraging destructive eating patterns.

There are two types of carbohydrate, or "carb", that we need to concern ourselves with. Simply put, these are slow-releasing carbs and fast-releasing carbs.

● The slow-releasing carbs are complex carbohydrates – these are "the good guys". They are principally brown or green foods with all their fibre intact. The fibre slows down the release of energy, which means that these foods sustain our energy levels.

● Fast-releasing carbs are "the bad guys". They include refined white starchy foods, sugars and alcohol, which have lost most of their integral fibre. As a result, they give us a quick "hit" of energy followed by an energy dip.

The carbohydrate list opposite gives an overview and can be memorized as a quick guide. But the effects of foods are more complex than this, and more information is given in the Glycaemic Index Chart on page 64. The glycaemic index is a list of carbohydrate foods and their energy-releasing potential. All foods are measured against glucose, which

scores 100. Glucose is a sugar that provides instant energy for our cells to use – it goes straight into the bloodstream and does not have to be digested or processed in any way.) This may sound like a good thing, and indeed in recent decades, athletes have used it before a race to give themselves a quick burst of energy. However, we now know that this is not very helpful, because while their energy levels will soar very quickly, this is immediately followed by a severe energy dip, when blood sugar plummets.

When blood sugar is low, the brain is not able to function properly, and we feel sleepy, confused or even faint. The body goes into crisis, which stresses it further. To conserve energy levels, and guard any remaining glucose in the bloodstream for critical brain functions, the body overwhelms us with a need to lie down, or close our eyes. As discussed earlier, fast-releasing sugars have a fundamental effect on brain chemicals and stress hormones.

Insulin resistance is another problem triggered by excessive consumption of carbohydrates. Individuals with this problem

CARBOHYDRATES AT A GLANCE

"GOOD GUYS" – SLOW-RELEASE COMPLEX CARBOHYDRATES WITH FIBRE INTACT

Wholemeal bread

Brown rice

Wholewheat pasta

Porridge oats

Jacket potato

Vegetables

Fruit

"BAD GUYS" – FAST-RELEASE CARBOHYDRATES WITH MOST FIBRE REMOVED

White or "brown" (not wholemeal) bread

White rice

White pasta

Instant oats

Mashed or boiled potato (no skin)

Sugar

Alcohol

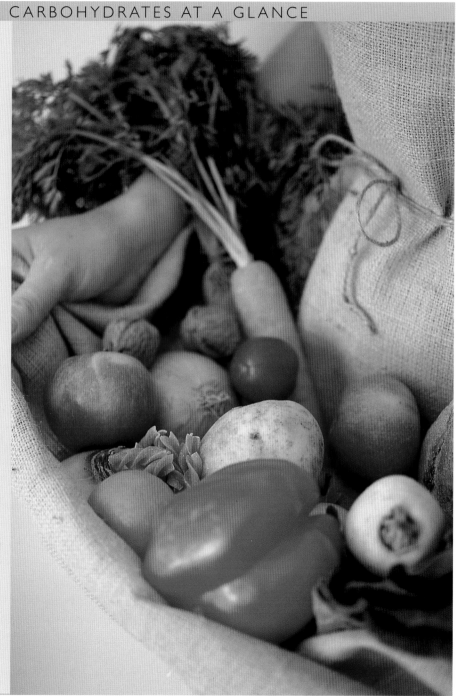

SIGNS OF BLOOD SUGAR IMBALANCE

- Do you need more than eight hours sleep a night, or are you slow to wake up in the morning?
- Do you often feel drowsy during the day?
- Do you sometimes lose concentration?
- Do you have less energy than you used to?
- Do you need something to get you going in the morning, or to boost flagging energy during the day (tea, coffee, sugar, cigarettes)?
- Are you addicted to sweet foods?
- Do you suffer from carbohydrate cravings?
- Do you get dizzy, irritable or shaky if you do not eat often?
- Do you have any addictions?
- Do you get excessively thirsty?

If you answer "yes" four times or more, you may need to address blood sugar balance.

SWEET DISGUISE

Sugar goes under a number of aliases on food packaging. Here are some of the names to look for:

Sugars	Bulk sweeteners	Artificial sweeteners
Sucrose		
Glucose	Sorbitol	Aspartame
Malt	Xylitol	Acesulfame K
Honey	Mannitol	Saccharine
Dextrose	Isomalt	Nutrasweet™
Maltose		
Lactose		

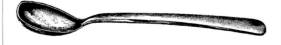

have high levels of insulin in the blood, which has been brought about by their high level of blood sugar. However, their cells have become resistant to the effects of the insulin, and are therefore unable to use the blood sugar for energy, so insulin levels remain high. People with insulin resistance often find that they have difficulty losing weight, because as the blood sugar is unable to be used efficiently for energy, it is stored in fat cells instead. Their diet needs to be revised to include a better mix of proteins and complex carbohydrates, as discussed a little later in the book.

One of the more serious problems linked to a cycle of blood sugar peaks and troughs, and particularly to insulin resistance, is that it harms body tissues. This is called glycosylation damage and for people suffering from diabetes, it can lead to serious problems with the eyes, cardiovascular system and kidneys. For people who experience blood sugar control problems, but do not go on to develop diabetes, glycosylation damage is associated with many degenerative diseases, including cardiovascular health problems, arthritis and Alzheimer's disease.

Eating too much sugar and refined carbohydrates also causes a mineral, chromium, to be excreted in the urine. This is detrimental because it is needed to help regulate blood sugar. Chromium is an important component of a substance produced in the liver, called glucose tolerance factor, which helps insulin to work properly. Because of these varied effects, the consumption of sugar and refined carbohydrates can have devastating consequences for the body if they are eaten to excess over a long period of time.

Sugar is the number one addictive substance in our diets. Food manufacturers are well aware of the dependency it encourages, and it is put into virtually every processed or packaged food. This sugar accounts for a massive 80 per cent of the 45–68kg (100–150lb) of sugar each one of us consumes annually – 36 teaspoonsful a day. And these figures exclude the sugar absorbed through alcohol consumption, which is another major source.

You need to become a sleuth to uncover the presence of sugar in the foods you eat. Of course, foods such as chocolate, biscuits, cookies, sweet pastries, candy and sweets are all obvious sources of sugar. But do you realize that breakfast cereals, hamburger buns, ready-made sauces, yoghurt and savoury snacks all contain sugar as well? All these sugary foods have a cumulative effect.

Many people resort to artificial sweeteners in order to avoid sugar. Manufacturers also routinely load processed foods with them, particularly since sweeteners are much cheaper than sugar. The problem with sweeteners, apart from the risk of toxicity and the need for the body to process and eliminate these useless chemicals, is that they do nothing to quell the desire for sweet foods and sugar. It is better, on balance, to retrain your taste buds by slowly reducing the amount of sugar in your diet, replacing it with naturally sweet sources of carbohydrates such as fruit.

HIDDEN SUGAR

The amount of sugar contained in food may surprise you. Here are some examples:

PRODUCT	ROUNDED TSP SUGAR	PRODUCT	ROUNDED TSP SUGAR
Digestive biscuits (1 biscuit)	½	Baked beans (½ medium tin)	2½
Chocolate digestive biscuits (1 biscuit)	1	Hot night-time drink (3 tsp powder mix)	1-2
Madeira cake (1 slice)	4	Cola (1 can)	8
Fruit-flavoured yoghurt (1 small carton)	4½	Chocolate (150g/5oz) bar)	8
Jam (2 tsp)	2½	Fruit gums (1 small pack)	2
Ice-cream (1 scoop)	2	Mints (1 small tube)	7½
Cornflakes (3 tbsp)	½	Hamburger bun (1 bun)	1
Muesli (1½ tbsp)	1½	Crisps (1 small bag)	½
Puffed wheat cereal (3 tbsp)	4	Tinned sweetcorn	2
Tinned/packet soup (½ tin/ ¼ packet)	½–1	Tomato ketchup (2 tsp)	½

It's a funny thing about life; if you refuse to accept anything but the best, you very often get it.

W. SOMERSET MAUGHAM

Glycaemic index chart

Use this chart to discover the glycaemic score of carbohydrate foods, which measures their energy-releasing potential. The foods are measured against glucose, with a score of 100. This is a type of sugar that when eaten, goes straight into the bloodstream without being digested or processed: it instantly sends blood sugar sky-high. Foods with a low glycaemic index release sugar into the bloodstream slowly, and are therefore better for you (in terms of blood sugar levels) than foods with a high glycaemic index, which make blood sugar levels soar.

LOW GLYCAEMIC FOODS

Foods to enjoy without worrying about their effect on blood sugar levels are those with a glycaemic score of under 50.

Sugars and sweet foods
Orange juice*	50
Apple juice*	38
Chocolate (70% cocoa solids)	22
Fructose (in moderation)	22

Whole fruit
Oranges	44
Plums	39
Apples	38
Pears	37
Dried apricots	31
Grapefruit	25
Stewed fruit (no sugar)	25
Cherries	22

Breads and crackers
Pumpernickel bread	50
Mixed grain bread	48

Grain products
Brown rice	50
Wholewheat pasta	37
Barley	31

Cereals
Whole porridge oats	49
All bran	42
Rice bran	19

Pulses
Baked beans	48
Baked beans (sugar free)	40
Chickpeas	36
Blackeye beans	33
Butter beans	31
Haricot beans	31
Lentils	29
Soya beans	14

Dairy products
Ice-cream (in moderation)	50
Milk, skimmed	32
Milk, whole	27
Yoghurt, plain	14

Vegetables
Sweet potato (cooked)	50
Sweetcorn	50
Carrot (raw)	49
Peas	48
Most other vegetables	10–20

Snacks and drinks
Peanuts	14
Nuts and seeds	14
Tomato or vegetable juice	12

* Use as a sweetener, dilute 50/50 with water to drink

HIGH GLYCAEMIC FOODS

Foods with a glycaemic score of between 51 and 70 can be enjoyed in moderation. Avoid, as much as possible, most foods that score between 71 and 100. (Fruits and vegetables, however, are important sources of vitamins and minerals.) When carbohydrates are processed, it generally increases their glycaemic index – maize scores 70, but cornflakes are 83. Remember that it is how you eat a food that counts. A small portion of a vegetable with a higher glycaemic score, eaten as part of a main meal, will have much less of an effect on blood sugar levels than a bar of sugary chocolate eaten on its own.

Sugars

Maltose (beer)	105
Glucose	100
Chocolate, milk	68
Sugar, white or brown (sucrose)	64
Honey/jam	58

Fruit

Watermelon	72
Pineapple	66
Melon	65
Raisins	64
Grapes	60
Dried fruit (most)	60
Bananas	54
Kiwi fruit	53

Breads and crackers

French baguette	95
White or "brown" bread	78
Rice cakes	77
Bagel	72
Wholemeal bread	69
Crumpet	69
Rye crackers	65
Oatcakes	54

Vegetables

Parsnips (cooked)	97
Carrots (cooked)	85
Potato (baked)	85
French fries	75
Beetroot (cooked)	64
Yams (cooked)	51

Grain products

White rice	72
Biscuits	70
Pastry	59
Basmati rice (white)	58
White pasta	55

Cereals

Cornflakes	83
Puffed rice	82
Wheat biscuits	70
Muesli	56
Bran flakes	54

Snacks and drinks

Alcohol	80–100
Corn chips	74
Colas and similar	68
Fruit squash (diluted)	66
Muesli bar	61
Potato crisps (high in fat)	54

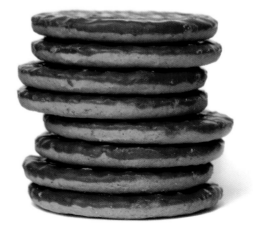

Protein power

When aiming to protect yourself from the effects of stress, it is particularly important to include proteins in the diet, because they have an important role to play in balancing the effects of carbohydrates. We need proteins for building and repairing body issues, and for producing hormones, enzymes and nerve chemicals. They are also vital for maintaining a healthy immune system. Someone who has been under severe stress for a long time will have a suppressed immune system, and may require extra protein.

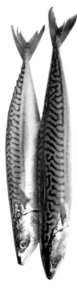

AMINO ACIDS

The structure of a protein is rather like a chain made up of links called amino acids. We require 22 amino acids, eight of which are termed essential, because our bodies cannot manufacture them. If we consume these eight, the body is able to make the remaining 14 and many more besides.

The foods that give us the eight essential amino acids we need, in perfect balance, are animal proteins: meat, poultry, fish, eggs, milk, yoghurt and cheese. Plant proteins also supply amino acids, though not all eight in one food. Protein-rich plant sources include soya, mycoprotein (mushrooms), beans, lentils, peas and legumes, fresh nuts and fresh seeds. A varied vegetarian diet of complementary foods, such as lentil curry and rice, or pasta and vegetables, will provide the full complement of essential amino acids. (This is not strictly necessary, as we have a pool of amino acids in our bodies for use when needed, however it is helpful, if you are a vegetarian or vegan, to know how to get the best out of proteins when planning meals.)

Many of us eat too much protein. In the West, it is common to have a meal consisting of a huge piece of meat with a meagre amount of vegetables. An excess of protein is damaging, because it has to be detoxified and eliminated, as has any excess. However, many people go to the other extreme and typically eat meals consisting mainly of refined carbohydrates with little protein, for example a bowl of spaghetti with a tomato sauce, or toast with jam or honey for breakfast. This leads to problems with insulin balance, and is not helpful for supporting the adrenal hormones.

INSULIN AND GLUCAGON

Diets based on the principles of "food combining" have become very popular in recent years. These involve eating proteins and carbohydrates at separate meals, and they are most suitable for people with digestive problems. However, it is a scientific fact that eating the two food groups in the same meal has a regulating effect on the hormones controlling blood sugar, insulin and glucagon, as well as on the adrenal hormones. People who are under a lot of stress need to make sure that they combine complex carbohydrates with proteins. Carbohydrates trigger insulin, while proteins regulate the effects of insulin by bringing the opposing

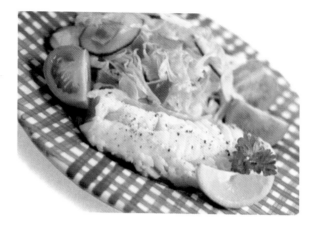

hormone, glucagon, into play. It is easy to understand how to avoid an insulin–blood sugar roller-coaster when you compare their effects (see chart).

In order to keep our energy levels constant, and to avoid the wild ups and downs that stress hormones can have on our blood sugar levels, we need to maintain a balance between insulin and glucagon. From the chart it would be easy to assume that, in addition to the medium-protein complex-carb meal, protein-only or high-protein low-carbohydrate meals are the most balanced. However, it would be exceedingly unhealthy to eat only high-protein meals. If the protein came from meat, there would be a high amount of saturated fats and no fibre. An excess of any sort of protein (especially in the absence of other regulating dietary factors) would stress the kidneys and liver. Also, a surfeit of proteins would

stimulate metabolic activity during processing by the body, causing more stress, and could contribute to osteoporosis by leaching calcium out of the bones (the acid residue left behind by proteins needs to be alkalized using calcium).

The best solution to the meal problem is to eat proteins together with a good amount of vegetables and fruits, which have little effect on blood sugar balance (see the Glycaemic Index Chart on page 64), or to eat small amounts of complex carbohydrates with roughly equal quantities of proteins. It is detrimental to eat large amounts of refined carbohydrates, which raise insulin levels dramatically.

BALANCING BLOOD SUGAR

It is not necessary for everybody to take steps to balance their blood sugar levels: it depends on a number of factors such as the type of diet eaten for the preceding few years, body type, genetics, and whether there is insulin resistance. However, the majority of people who feel that they have been under stress for a while will probably have edged towards blood sugar imbalance, because of the intimate relationship between adrenaline, insulin and glucagon. If this sounds like you, the chances are that by increasing protein levels in relation to carbohydrates, it will make a significant difference, especially if you habitually eat meals and snacks that are high in carbohydrates, or use stimulating drinks and foods to keep yourself going throughout the day.

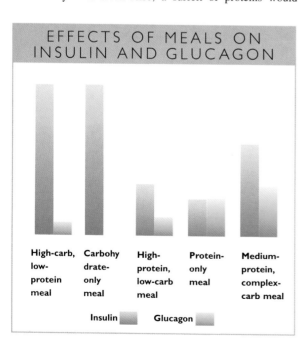

EFFECTS OF MEALS ON INSULIN AND GLUCAGON

High-carb, low-protein meal	Carbohydrate-only meal	High-protein, low-carb meal	Protein-only meal	Medium-protein, complex-carb meal

Insulin ▮   Glucagon ▮

Energy meal choices

The best meals to sustain energy, promote brain function and support adrenal performance are those that contain complex carbohydrates (C) in a balance with proteins (P). It is also wise to bulk out meals with vegetables, salads and fruits as often as possible – also designated (C). Here are some ideas.

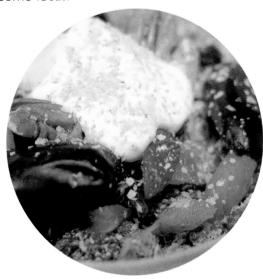

BREAKFAST

■ Wholemeal toast (C) with poached egg (P) and grilled tomatoes (C).

■ Plain live yoghurt (P) with chopped fruit (C) and ground sunflower seeds (P).

■ Sugar-free muesli (C) with chopped fruit (C), soya or dairy milk (P) and ground pumpkin seeds (P).

■ Yoghurt (P) – try goat's yoghurt for a change – with wholegrain rice puffs (C) and berries (C).

■ Lean grilled bacon (P) with mushrooms, onions and tomatoes (C).

LIGHT MEALS

■ Mixed green herb salad (C) with a small amount of crumbled feta cheese (P) and walnuts (P).

■ Baked jacket potato (C) filled with sweetcorn (C) and salmon (P) bound with houmous (P/C). Serve with fresh coleslaw (C).

■ Thick lentil (P) and vegetable (C) soup.

■ Beans (P) on rye toast (C).

■ Tempeh or chicken burger (P) with shredded Chinese cabbage (C) sprinkled with soya sauce and sesame seeds (P) on a wholemeal bun (C).

■ Sardines (P) on wholemeal toast (C) and tomato salad (C).

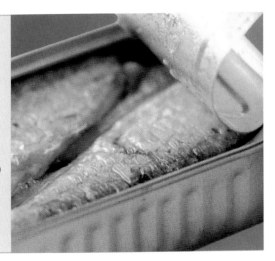

MAIN MEALS

■ Flaked smoked fish (P) with brown rice (C), onions and peas (P/C).

■ Beans (P) in spicy tomato, garlic and onion sauce with wholemeal cous-cous (C).

■ Wholewheat pasta (C) or buckwheat noodles (C), with mushroom and seafood (P) sauce.

■ Refried beans (P) and tacos (C) with guacamole and salsa.

■ Salad niçoise with tuna (P), egg (P), green beans, olives, millet (C) and herb olive oil dressing.

■ Roast turkey (P) with broccoli or other vegetables, roasted whole baby potatoes (C) and whole garlic cloves.

■ Chicken (P) and coriander curry with brown rice (C).

■ Grilled salmon fillets (P) with green beans (C) and savoury quinoa (C/P).

■ Tofu (P) stir-fried with julienned vegetables (C) and ginger, served with brown rice (C).

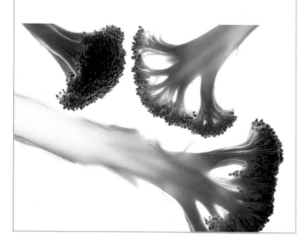

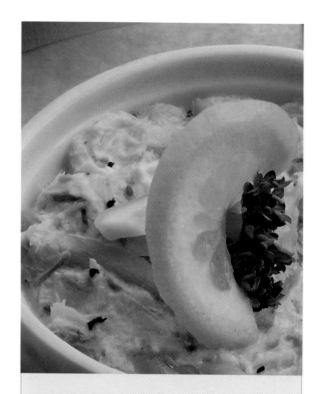

SNACKS

■ Rye crackers (C) spread with mackerel paté (P) and chopped cucumber.

■ Oatcakes (C) with nut butter (P) and strawberry slices (C).

■ Toast made from sprouted wheat bread (C) with tahini (P) and tomato (C).

■ Fruit (C) and nut (P) mix.

■ Grilled mozzarella (P) and pasta tomato sauce, on halved wholewheat pitta bread pockets (C).

■ Rice cakes (C) topped with cottage cheese (P) and sliced apple (C).

The fat factor

Fats have had a bad press and many health problems have been blamed on them – not least of all excess weight. They are the most energy-rich source of calories in our diet, providing nine calories per gram, compared to the four calories per gram contained in proteins and carbohydrates.

We tend to consume too many saturated and hydrogenated fats from sources such as meat, dairy products, margarine, cooking oils and packaged foods. And these are the kind of fats that sit on our hips and around our middles.

But certain fats are needed for good health – for building cell membranes in every cell in the body, for ensuring that the nervous system functions properly, and for making hormones. Chronic stress can be exacerbated if we do not provide the building blocks for the very hormones that are needed to deal with it. These building blocks are "healthy" fats, or polyunsaturated fats, (omega-3, omega-6, and omega-9), which can be found in the food below:

Omega-9 fats
Olive oil, avocados.
Omega-6 fats
Cold-pressed oils: sunflower, sesame, walnut.
Very fresh unroasted and unsalted nuts and seeds.
Grains, vegetables and their oils, corn oil, wheatgerm oil.
evening primrose oil, starflower oil, raspberry seed oil.
Omega-3 fats
Oily fish: mackerel, sardines, tuna, salmon, pilchards, anchovies, shark, pink trout and so on. Cold-pressed flax oil, linseeds, pumpkin seeds, walnuts, soya beans and hemp seeds.

Another good reason to include omega-6 and omega-3 fats in your diet is that they include the essential fatty acids which help to reduce inflammation. Conversely, saturated and

BETTER FAT CHOICES

INSTEAD OF	CHOOSE
Cooking oil (corn or sunflower oil)	Olive oil
Margarine	A scrape of butter
Butter	See the choices in "Spreads For Your Bread"
Cream	Greek yoghurt, low-fat yoghurt, Quark, tofu, soya cream
Full-fat milk	Skimmed milk, soya milk, oat milk or rice milk
Red meat (pork, lamb, beef)	Fish, organic skinless chicken or turkey, tofu, other soya products

SPREADS FOR YOUR BREAD

There are many substitutes that can be used instead of butter or margarine.

- Mackerel paté
- Salsa
- Olive oil mixed with minced garlic
- Houmous
- Tahini
- 100 per cent fruit jam
- Guacamole
- Nut butter
- Mushroom paté
- Vegetable paté

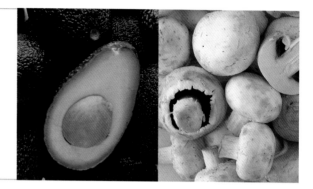

hydrogenated fats can make inflammation worse. When someone is under chronic pressure, the process of wound healing often becomes less efficient, and pre-existing inflammatory conditions such as arthritis, eczema or asthma may get worse. Part of the reason for this is that overtaxed adrenal glands do not have the physical reserves to pump out sufficient natural steroid hormones, which are designed to bring inflammation down. Many people then resort to asking their doctor for steroid creams or other medication. However, it is far better to boost your own reserves of natural steroid hormones by ensuring that adequate nutrient levels are maintained, and that the majority of the fats you eat are the essential fatty acids responsible for reducing inflammation. The body turns these into substances called PGE1 and PGE3, which oppose another substance called PGE2 promoted by animal fats. Hydrogenated fats (found in margarine and processed foods) cause inflammation, because they interfere with the conversion of healthy fats into PGE1 and PGE3.

Healthy fats have other benefits, especially in relation to the cardiovascular system. Stress causes the blood to thicken during the fight or flight response, in preparation for any injury that may occur. Many studies have shown that the omega-3 essential fatty acids have a blood-thinning effect that enhances cardiovascular health.

FAST FOOD CHOICES

INSTEAD OF	CHOOSE
A bacon or cheese sandwich.	A huge avocado, tomato and spring onion sandwich on wholemeal or rye bread.
A hamburger at a burger bar.	A flame-grilled chicken burger or a bean burger in a roll with salad. Skip the fries.
A hunk of cheese and cream crackers.	Houmous on rye crackers with celery.
A doner kebab.	Falafel or chicken kebab in a pitta pocket, with salad and tahini dressing.
A four-cheese and salami pizza.	Pizza topped with prawns or tuna, onion, peppers, mushrooms and olives. Skip the cheese (or ask for less) and double the tomato to keep it moist.
Fried rice and fried noodles.	Stir-fried Chinese vegetables and broccoli, king prawns in ginger, steamed rice.
A savoury pie and french fries.	A baked potato with tuna filling (go easy on the mayonnaise) and salad.

Antioxidant shields

Antioxidants are wonderful things. Imagine that we are constantly under fire from millions of little arrows called free radicals, which cause oxidation damage in the body. Antioxidants are shields that protect us from them. When cells are damaged by free radicals, they cannot function properly. This type of damage is partly responsible for a wide range of illnesses, including all the degenerative diseases such as arthritis, cardiovascular disease, Alzheimer's and cancer.

Free radicals are unstable molecules which, in an effort to stabilize themselves, steal electrons from any available place, such as our body tissues. External sources of free radicals include the sun, bonfires, barbecues, cigarettes, car exhausts and hydrogenated fats found in margarines and cooking oils. Free radicals are also created internally, by basic body processes such as breathing and digestion.

Antioxidants are heroic little molecules that kindly sacrifice themselves to spare us from giving up electrons from our cells. The more antioxidants we get in our diets, the better we are able to avoid the effects of free radicals. The main sources of antioxidants are fruits and vegetables. You may be convinced that antioxidants are good things, and that a diet high in fruits and vegetables is highly beneficial. But what does all this have to do with stress, and how do antioxidants form part of a stress protection plan?

Stress is one of the greatest internal sources of free radicals. This means that when we are stressed, increased damage to our body tissues takes place (quite possibly more than we are naturally able to protect ourselves from). When we are under prolonged stress, we succumb to more infections, pre-existing conditions worsen, and we are more susceptible to heart disease, stroke and cancer.

Stress increases free-radical damage by playing havoc with blood sugar levels. It also reduces the effectiveness of the anti-inflammatory hormones, and when inflammation is rampant it whips up a hot-bed of free-radical activity. Possible signs of inflammation include poor wound healing, wind, loose stools, arthritis, gastritis, chronic acne, eczema or psoriasis. Antioxidants can improve all of these. Beware of two other sources of free radicals, which we are more likely to consume when under stress: cigarettes and alcohol.

Set me a task in which I can put something of myself,

and it is a task no longer, it is a joy, it is art.

BLISS CARMEN

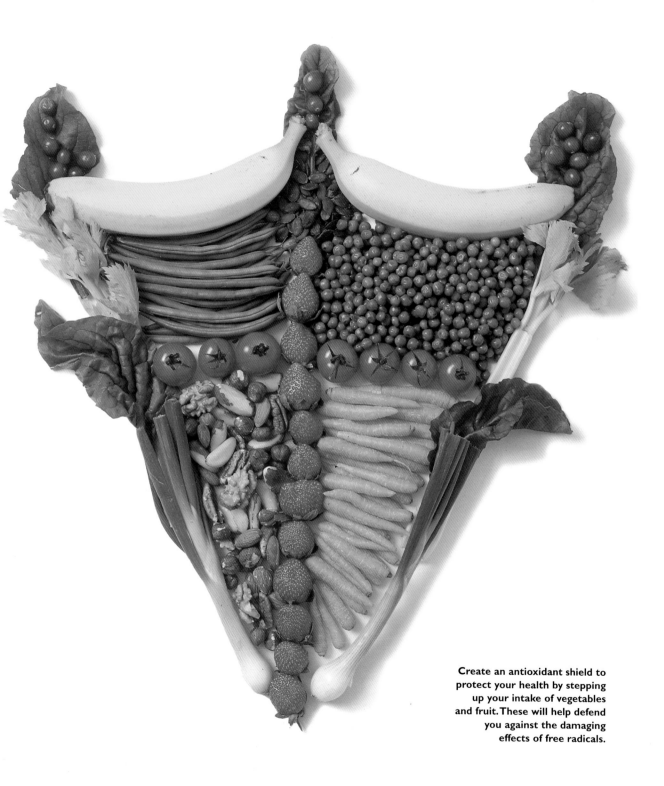

Create an antioxidant shield to protect your health by stepping up your intake of vegetables and fruit. These will help defend you against the damaging effects of free radicals.

Stress-busting superfoods

Some foods help to protect our bodies from the ravages of chronic stress by providing antioxidants and injecting a boost of concentrated nutrients. Plants contain phytochemicals, which are designed to protect them against the stresses that nature throws at them – radiation from the sun, viruses, bacteria and parasites. When we eat these plants, the benefits are transferred to us. The following pages are a colour-coded tour of the protection that foods offer.

PINK AND RED

GRAPEFRUIT	PRAWNS	RED GRAPES	RED ONIONS	REDBUSH TEA
These colourful citrus fruits contain lycopene, as well as loads of bioflavonoids. The sour taste of grapefruit increases the flow of digestive juices and helps the digestion of meat. Serve them at the end of a meal to refresh the palate. Grapefruit seed extract is a powerful anti-bacterial agent.	Pretty in pink, these little sea gems are valuable sources of selenium, zinc and iodine, which help to maintain our defensive antioxidant enzymes, repair tissues and regulate the thyroid, which governs metabolism. Keep some handy in the freezer as they are ideal for a boost of nutrients in salads or stir-frys.	The anthocyanins contained in red grapes shield them from the sun's radiation, and can do the same for us. They also help to save our skin from the impact of stress. Red wine has the same benefits; however, to avoid the negative effects of alcohol, you could substitute red grape juice!	All the onion family contain the potent antioxidant quercitin, but red onions are a more concentrated source of it. Quercitin, along with the sulphur amino acids also in onions, helps to excrete toxic heavy-metal compounds that build up in the body. Onions also have antibiotic, antiviral and anti-candida (*Candida albicans*, a yeast-like fungus) properties.	Drunk in southern Africa for centuries, where it is known as rooibos, this tea is an excellent source of phenol antioxidants. It also provides sufficient fluoride to protect teeth without some of the enzyme-inhibiting effects of the type of fluoride in toothpaste, which has been shown to suppress immune and thyroid function, and interfere with bone cell turnover.

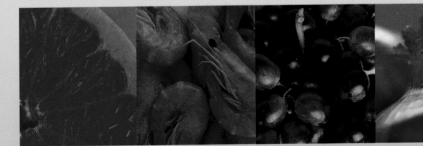
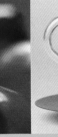
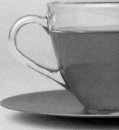

TOMATOES	ROSEHIPS	CHERRIES	WATERMELON	RED PEPPERS
Tomatoes are the richest source of lycopene, a valuable antioxidant that is more potent than beta-carotene. Research has shown that eating 10 servings a week gives significant protection against some cancers. Interestingly, cooked tomatoes provide a more concentrated source of lycopene than raw tomatoes, as cooking helps to release the lycopene for absorption. Tomatoes also contain carotenoids, vitamin C and quercitin. Raise your intake with tomato salad, tinned tomatoes, sun-dried tomatoes, tomato sauces and soups.	These are the shiny red fruit left behind after the roses have blossomed. They are extremely concentrated sources of antioxidants, as well containing lots of vitamin C, flavonoids, tannins and mucilages. They are good for maintaining immune health and healthy collagen and fighting gastric inflammation and diarrhoea. Look in a healthfood store for rosehip tea or a cordial, which will help to ward off many bugs in winter. Rosehip soup is popular in Sweden.	Cherries contain anthocyanins, potent antioxidants which particularly protect the respiratory tract. Cherries also contain a painkilling compound, and 20 cherries are equal in effect to one aspirin! All edible red berries, such as raspberries and strawberries, also contain these valuable anthocyanins. These fruit are also excellent sources of vitamin C, quercitin and lignans, all of which are also antioxidants.	This juicy fruit gives us plenty of lycopene, and its seeds are very rich in potassium. Next time you pick up a slice of watermelon, eat both flesh and seeds for maximum nutrients. The seeds are crunchy and taste really good. Potassium is important for brain function, water balance and blood pressure control and eliminating toxins. When you make watermelon juice include some of the (scrubbed) rind for its silicon (good for hair and nails) and for blood-building chlorophyll. Watermelon juice is the ideal source of mineral-rich distilled water.	Peppers are a concentrated source of the all-important vitamin C, and contain more of this stress-busting vitamin than citrus fruit. Red, yellow and orange peppers are good sources of carotenoids, the family of compounds to which beta-carotene belongs. Enjoy peppers raw, stuffed, roasted, or chopped into sauces and stews. Its hot cousin, the chilli pepper, is a wonderful blood cleanser and detoxifier when used in moderation.

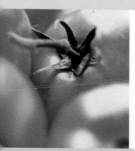
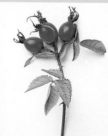
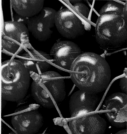
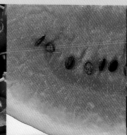
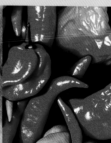

BLUE, PURPLE AND BROWN

BLACKBERRIES	AUBERGINE	FIGS AND DATES	MOLASSES	NUTS AND SEEDS
Blackberries are packed with antioxidant nutrients, including the powerful proanthocyanins, which is why a hot blackcurrant drink has been used for centuries to keep colds and infections at bay. 25 years ago, Finland had the highest heart disease mortality rate in the world. The Finns introduced a health campaign which highlighted eating berries and have since seen a 50 per cent drop in the death rate.	This is a versatile vegetable and it is particularly good grilled or roasted with peppers, onion and garlic. Its rich range of nutrients includes calcium, magnesium, iron and folic acid. It is a member of the belladonna or nightshade family, which means that it may be unsuitable for people with arthritis. Do not cook aubergine in too much oil as it ends up too greasy; it is just as delicious cooked in very little oil.	Figs have a mild laxative effect, and contain an enzyme which helps to cleanse the digestive tract. Whether dried or fresh, they are high in fibre, and a good source of minerals, including magnesium, iron, copper and manganese. These are needed for the body's own built-in antioxidant systems. Because of their natural sweetness, dates are used as a sweetener in many health foods. As they contain vitamin B5, they are particularly beneficial if you are stressed.	Molasses is a residue from the process of refining sugar. It is exceptionally rich in B-vitamins and minerals, particularly iron and calcium. Molasses contains, weight for weight, more calcium than milk! Previous generations must have had a good idea of its high mineral content, because it was given to children, along with disgusting-tasting sulphur, to encourage a strong constitution. Molasses taste very sweet.	Fresh nuts and seeds are one of our most important sources of linoleic and linolenic acid, which are essential fatty acids. These are required for the membranes of each of the millions of cells that make up our body. Seeds contain about 20–30 per cent protein and also provide a source of calcium and magnesium in an ideal ratio for bone health. By sprouting seeds, their nutrient content can be increased by up to 200 per cent.

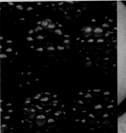
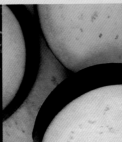
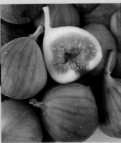
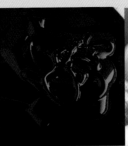
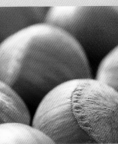

JUNIPER BERRIES

The mention of juniper berries may spur your thoughts towards a refreshing gin and tonic. Although possibly the most appealing way to consume juniper berries it is not, sadly, the best way of reaping all their benefits. In addition to their calming properties and ability to relax tired muscles, juniper berries, like many berries, are high in vitamin C and proanthocyanins. Add the berries to sweet or savoury dishes, or use them to make sauces.

CHOCOLATE

You may be surprised to see this on a list of superfoods! Chocolate is much maligned because the sugar content in most brands of chocolate makes it a nutritional disaster área. However, good-quality organic chocolate that is 70 per cent cocoa is sufficiently high in magnesium, calcium and polyphenol antioxidants to make it an acceptable treat from time to time, providing that the caffeine content is not a problem for you.

RYE

Rye is rarely refined, and so its mineral content remains high, and it has a rich flavour when made into bread. Its gluten content is less than that of wheat, and it is often better tolerated by those who are wheat sensitive. Like all whole grains, rye is a good source of B-vitamins. Whole rye has up to five times more fibre than most other whole grains and is excellent for stabilizing blood sugar. Rye flakes make a nutritious addition to mueslies and the grains can be sprouted to increase their nutrient value.

PURPLE SAGE

This is a delicious herb to add to salads, fish and meat dishes. It can also be made into a tea. Purple sage helps to bring down inflammation and is particularly good for respiratory problems. It also calms the digestive tract. This herb has been used to improve low moods, confusion and poor memory.

LIVER

Liver is one of the most concentrated sources of nutrients available to us. In addition to protein, carbohydrate and fat, it is packed with a whole range of essential vitamins and minerals. The liver is an animal's organ of detoxification, however, so choose organic meat, as it is less likely to be loaded up with pesticides and drugs.

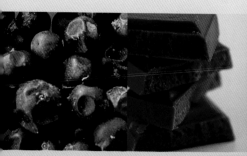
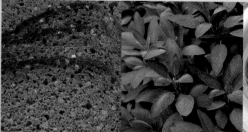
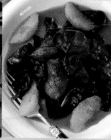

YELLOW AND ORANGE

EVENING PRIMROSE	EGG YOLKS	MANGOES	ORANGES/LEMONS	PAPAYA
Evening primrose oil is often taken as a supplement to counter premenstrual syndrome, and for eczema, acne and arthritis. This plant is one of the most concentrated sources of gamma-linoleic acid (GLA), which is needed for healthy sexual function and is highly anti-inflammatory. Stress, smoking and alcohol can prevent the efficient manufacture of GLA in the body, which is why people who are stressed often suffer from inflammation and why evening primrose oil can be so helpful in relieving it.	Much of the vitamin and mineral content of eggs depends on what the hen is fed on. Eggs are an excellent food, containing high amounts of vitamins A, D and E as well as some B-vitamins. Because eggs yolks contain fat and cholesterol, many people think that they should avoid them, yet cholesterol is required by the body to make hormones, including the stress-fighting steroid hormones.	Once you've mastered how to cut up a mango, cutting on either side of the stone (the less sticky method), mangoes are a great source of nutrients, particularly beta-carotene (between 300–3000mcg per 100gms of flesh), vitamin E, vitamin C, and minerals including iron. They are high in gallic acid which is helpful for bowel health. Mango juice can help with a fever and is cleansing for the blood.	Citrus fruits are well known for their vitamin C content, but they also boast almost all essential vitamins and minerals. Leave some of the white pith on the fruit as this is where most of the minerals are found, in addition to the valuable flavanoid, quercetin. Citrus fruits also contain pectin, which helps the body to eliminate toxins. The rind is a valuable source of limonene which is a powerful liver restorer and may have anti-cancer properties. If you use grated rind, make sure you use unwaxed, organic fruit.	A refreshing starter of papaya is a marvellous way to begin a meal. As well as being rich in the antioxidant vitamins A and C, and a source of minerals such as potassium, papayas contain an enzyme, papain, which helps to digest proteins. If the fruit is slightly unripe it contains more of this enzyme. It is also mildly antiseptic and healing, making papaya the tastiest way to heal mouth ulcers!

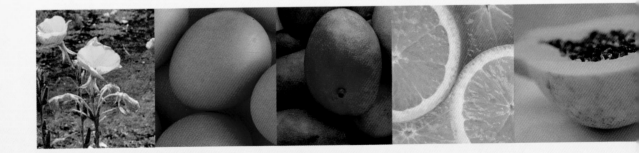

BANANAS	TURMERIC	SWEETCORN	PINEAPPLE	APRICOTS
Bananas are high in potassium, so they are good for keeping potassium levels topped up during periods of stress. Ripe bananas are also great for digestive health and can help diarrhoea and constipation, although ironically, some people cannot digest bananas well. A banana is about 80–100 kilocalories, making it a healthy, low-calorie snack. They are made up, almost totally, of carbohydrate. Avoid eating more than one a day if you have blood sugar balance problems, because they have a high glycaemic index.	Used as a yellow colouring and spice in Indian cuisine, the active constituent, curcumin, its yellow pigment, is a powerful anti-inflammatory and antioxidant. It also has anti-cancer properties. Turmeric stimulates liver enzymes and bile flow, and is used to treat jaundice. It is highly protective against environmental pollutants.	Sweetcorn is not a vegetable, but a grain, and is 80 per cent carbohydrate. It was first cultivated by Native Americans, but later became popular in Mexico, where the tortilla was born. Its yellow colour reveals it to be rich in beta-carotene and vitamin A. Unlike other grains, it is also a fairly good source of vitamin C. Baby corn is high in folic acid. As well as the more familiar cornflakes, sweetcorn and popcorn, experiment with tortillas and corn bread.	Pineapple contains the digestive enzyme bromelain, so it is a great accompaniment to a savoury meal, and excellent for sweet and sour dishes. Pineapples are rich in vitamins A and C, potassium, calcium and the important minerals selenium and manganese, which are needed to protect our cells and tissues from oxidation damage. The best way to test the fruit for ripeness is to see if you can easily pull a leaf from its crown – if you can, it is ripe.	These are one of the staple foods of the Hunzas people, who are well known for their longevity. Apricots are especially rich in beta-carotene, which can be made into vitamin A in the body, and fairly high in vitamin C. They also contain zinc, which is one of the vital anti-stress nutrients. Dried apricots, together with a handful of fresh nuts, make a good, energy-balanced snack. Choose unsulphured dried fruit.

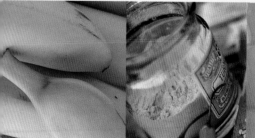
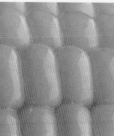
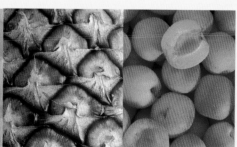

Vitamins and minerals

Vitamins and minerals have particular uses for supporting the body against stress, but no single nutrient works alone. For example, in food, magnesium will be present alongside calcium, zinc and boron, which help it to work effectively. These are called co-factors. A healthy diet is vital to obtain the full variety of nutrients necessary for the correct functioning of the body. If you use supplements, always take a multivitamin and multi-mineral capsule as well as specific nutrients, to help them work more efficiently. Do not exceed the doses printed on the packaging.

FOR NERVOUS STRESS			
NUTRIENT	FUNCTION	FOOD SOURCES	DAILY SUPPLEMENTS
B-COMPLEX	Used for energy and for the nervous system, muscles and heart. Vital for mental function. Used for adrenal glands and the stress response mechanism.	Wholegrains, oatmeal, legumes, dried yeast, liver, yoghurt, cottage cheese, lean meat, figs, dates, eggs, molasses, nuts, fish, green leafy vegetables, orange-coloured fruit (such as apricots, cantaloupe melon, pumpkin).	50–100mg. Best taken as a complex.
CALCIUM	Essential for nerve message transmission. Keeps the heart beating regularly.	Dairy products (well-absorbed from yoghurt), soya (such as tofu), nuts, seeds, dried beans, green leafy vegetables, broccoli, sardines, salmon.	300–500mg. Best taken with equal amount of magnesium.
IODINE	Regulates the thyroid gland, which is necessary for proper mental and metabolic function.	Kelp, samphire and other sea vegetables, all seafood, iodised salt.	Usually taken as a kelp supplement, or put seaweed granules in an empty salt mill to use as a condiment.
MAGNESIUM	Used for the stress response. Essential for nerve and muscle function. Needed for correct calcium usage.	Dark green leafy vegetables, citrus fruit, seeds, nuts, raisins, sweetcorn, mushrooms, garlic, onions, potatoes, chicken.	300–500mg.

FOR PHYSICAL STRESS			
NUTRIENT	FUNCTION	FOOD SOURCES	DAILY SUPPLEMENTS
VITAMIN A	Promotes healthy bones, teeth and gums. Needed to repair skin and mucous membranes (and so protects against respiratory and digestive infections). Antioxidant.	Full-fat dairy products, liver, cod-liver oil, oily fish, egg yolks.	7,500–20,000 ius (international units). Do not take if you think you may be pregnant – use beta-carotene instead.
VITAMIN C	Vital for the immune system (antiviral, antibacterial, used for white blood cell manufacture). Required for skin, bone and cartilage formation, and for wound healing. Used in large quantities during any period of stress. Antioxidant.	Citrus fruit, strawberries, kiwi fruit, cabbage, cauliflower, green leafy vegetables, peppers, potatoes, sweet potatoes, broccoli, beansprouts.	500mg–1g for maintenance; 1–3g if extra help needed.
VITAMIN D	Helps calcium to be utilized for bones, and works with vitamins A and C above.	Oily fish, egg yolks, dairy produce.	400 ius if regularly exposed to the sun, 800 ius if usually indoors.
VITAMIN E	Protects cell membranes. Helps to prevent scarring. Keeps blood from getting too thick (a by-product of stress). Antioxidant.	Wheatgerm, cold-pressed vegetable oils, green leafy vegetables, olive oil, eggs, soya beans, fresh nuts and seeds, wholegrains, brown rice, tomatoes.	100–1000 ius (caution if on blood-thinning medication).
VITAMIN K	Needed for blood clotting. Used for bone health.	Yoghurt, alfalfa, egg yolks, fish liver oils, green leafy vegetables, milk, safflower oil, kelp, raspberry leaf tea.	Not usually supplemented, though it is available.
MANGANESE	Used for thyroid (see iodine above) and for energy cycle.	Nuts, green leafy vegetables, peas, beets, egg yolks, wholegrain cereals.	5–50mg.
ZINC	Vital for all cell growth and repair. Necessary for immune system function and enzyme production.	Nuts and seeds, meat, eggs, sardines, wholegrains, tuna, brown rice, berries.	10–25 mg.

FOR ENVIRONMENTAL STRESS			
NUTRIENT	FUNCTION	FOOD SOURCES	DAILY SUPPLEMENTS
VITAMIN C	Helps to reduce histamine-related allergies. Escorts heavy metals (lead, aluminium, mercury, cadmium, arsenic) out of the body. Helps to lessen radiation-induced damage. Interferes with the conversion of nitrates into carcinogenic compounds. Antioxidant.	See page 81.	See page 81.
VITAMIN E	Protects against chlorine used in bleached products, water and pools.	See page 81.	See page 81.
BETA-CAROTENE	Strengthens mucous membranes against airborne allergens and toxins. Antioxidant. Converts into vitamin A.	Green leafy vegetables, orange-coloured vegetables and fruit (such as carrots, sweet potato, pumpkin and apricots).	5–20mg.
CALCIUM	A general antagonist to all the main heavy metals.	See page 80.	See page 80.
SELENIUM	Detoxifies mercury and arsenic. An antioxidant needed for one of the most important antioxidant and detoxification systems. Helps to protect against radiation-induced damage.	Wheatgerm, bran, rice, tomatoes, broccoli, brazil nuts, seafood.	100–200mcg. Do not exceed maximum dose as selenium can be toxic in excess.
ZINC	A general antagonist to all the main heavy metals. Helps to protect against radiation-induced damage. Antioxidant.	See page 81.	See page 81.

FOR NUTRITIONAL STRESS			
NUTRIENT	FUNCTION	FOOD SOURCES	DAILY SUPPLEMENTS
B-COMPLEX	Used for the energy cycle. Depleted by alcohol, tea, coffee, smoking, sugar, contraceptive pill, painkillers, antibiotics.	See page 80.	See page 80.
VITAMIN C	Used for energy and stress, but depleted by cooking, smoking and alcohol.	See page 81.	See page 81.
VITAMIN E	Destroyed by heat, freezing and food processing. Necessary if high amounts of processed foods and oils are consumed.	See page 81.	See page 81.
CHROMIUM	Excreted in the urine when a large amount of sugar is eaten. Needed to regulate insulin. Helps to lower cholesterol levels and to supply protein to where it is needed in the body.	Wholegrains, shellfish, brewer's yeast, brown rice, liver, eggs, lettuce, bananas, oranges, mushrooms, parsnips, apples, strawberries, potatoes.	100–500mcg.
IRON	Required to form red blood cells and used for the energy cycle. Often deficient as a result of a highly processed diet. Needed to metabolize B-vitamins.	Red meat, liver, egg yolks, dried fruit (such as apricots, raisins, figs, prunes), asparagus, kale, seaweed, oatmeal, walnuts, sunflower seeds, mushrooms.	10mg. Best taken with vitamin C-rich foods.
POTASSIUM	Needed for brain function and water balance. Deficiency likely if insufficient fresh food in the diet.	All vegetables and fruit, but particularly bananas, watermelon and potatoes.	Not usually supplemented.

How to eat a nutrient-rich diet

The food groups that are richest in the stress-fighting vitamins and minerals are grains, pulses, vegetables, nuts and seeds, fruits, lean meats and dairy produce.

GRAINS

Wholegrains satisfy hunger, provide energy, calm nerves, balance brain chemistry and encourage deep sleep. They also promote healthy elimination, good memory, clear thinking and quick reflexes. Our knowledge of grains tends to be limited to wheat, rice and oats. But there are many other interesting types to eat, such as rye, barley, corn, millet, spelt, tricale, buckwheat and quinoa.

BEANS AND PULSES

Many different types of beans and pulses are available and they can be added to soups, stews, pies and salads, eaten as a vegetable, or made into dips. Chickpeas, mung beans and most others are also good for sprouting. These mineral-rich vegetables are also good as a meat substitute. Enjoy lentil soup, houmous, home-made baked beans, three-bean salad, Mexican refried bean dishes, and curry made from chickpeas or other beans. Add green peas to omelettes, include black-eye beans or flageolet beans in salads, and serve lentil terrine as a starter. Look in ethnic cookery books for ideas for other dishes that use beans and pulses.

VEGETABLES

All vegetables are full of vitamins and minerals. Frozen vegetables are as good as fresh, but canned vegetables will have lost vitamins and enzymes. Every day, make sure you eat at least three portions from among the following: green leafy vegetables, salad vegetables, root vegetables, or vegetables that are red, yellow or orange.

NUTS AND SEEDS

Nature's takeaway foods, which are rich in essential fatty acids as well as zinc, calcium and magnesium. Nuts and seeds need to be eaten when they are as fresh as possible, which means buying them in small packs from shops with a high turnover. Keep them in the fridge until ready to eat.

GLOVE-COMPARTMENT GOODIES

In those moments when you are stuck in a slow-moving traffic jam, the temptation to pull over to buy something unhealthy to chew on can be overwhelming. What can you keep in your glove compartment to keep you on the straight and narrow? (The following suggestions are equally useful for carrying round with you, or keeping stashed in your desk drawer.)

- ■ A packet of oatcakes.
- ■ Small pack of unsalted, unroasted mixed nuts and raisins.
- ■ Chinese rice crackers.
- ■ A piece of luscious fruit.
- ■ Wholemeal bread sticks or pretzels.
- ■ 100 per cent fruit chewy bar.
- ■ Sunflower or pumpkin seeds.
- ■ A small jar of olives or pickles.
- ■ Some organic chocolate (70 per cent cocoa).

Seeds such as sunflower, sesame, pumpkin, hemp, flax and pine nuts are delicious to munch as a snack, but you can also chop them and sprinkle them on to a variety of sweet or savoury dishes before serving, or grind them and add to soups or cereals.

FRUIT

Fruit is the original fast food: just grab it and eat it. It is also one of the best ways to redress the balance between potassium and sodium in our bodies, which is vital when managing stress. Eat at least three portions daily.

LEAN MEATS, POULTRY AND FISH

The typical Western diet tends to include too much fatty meat. Meat is a valuable source of zinc, iron and some B-vitamins, but unfortunately, it also often comes with a heavy load of saturated fat. For this reason it is best to limit meat to one small portion a day and to trim off all the visible fat. Think of meat as a condiment to add flavour to a dish, rather than being the focus of the meal. Instead of red meat, opt for skinless organic chicken, or game (while this is red meat it has little saturated fat and is naturally organic, and you can choose from pheasant, partridge and venison, when in season). Fish (especially the oily fish such as mackerel, sardines, salmon and tuna) is an excellent alternative.

DAIRY PRODUCE

While dairy produce is rich in minerals and also supplies some fat-soluble vitamins, this is another food that we often eat too much of, and high consumption has been linked to a number of health complaints. The best dairy products are skimmed milk, live "bio" yoghurt, cottage cheese, goat's cheese and sheep's cheese. As an alternative to milk, there are various substitutes such as soya, oat and rice milks, many of which have been fortified with minerals in order to match those in cow's milk. These substitutes are free of the substances that lead to many intolerances.

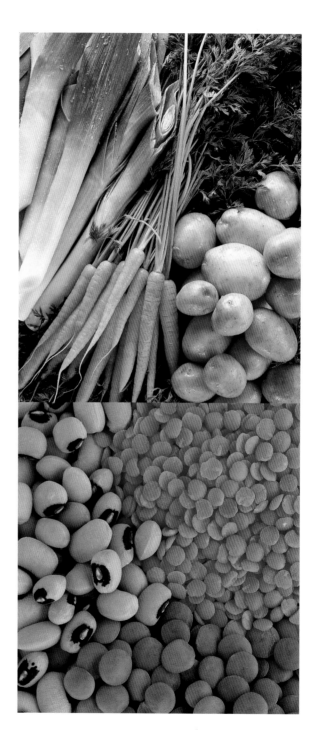

Stress-protection nutrients

If you are slightly overdrawn at the bank, you can cut back on spending in order to get back into credit. On the other hand, if you are seriously overdrawn, you need to apply different measures, together with resolving to build up reserves so that you don't go so far into the red again.

It is the same with maintaining a balance of nutrients in your body. If you are a little out of sorts, you can remedy it easily enough with a few dietary adjustments and some rest. If you overdo it, or if you know you will have a call on your reserves in the near future (you may be planning a family, going for a more ambitious job or just entering the winter months when you tend to get more colds), it may be a good idea to top up with some supplements.

Here we will look at the key stress protection nutrients, examining food sources and supplements. Of course, your overall health plan should encompass ensuring that you have a nutritious diet, making decisions that work for you, working on stress factors in your life, and just enjoying yourself more. But using nutritional supplements can be a boost when you need to get well as quickly as possible. The "adaptogens" are of particular interest. These are a number of ancilliary herbs and foods – ginseng, dong quai, royal jelly, and others – that have the ability to help the body to "adapt" to a new strain or stress, by stimulating the body's own mechanisms. The following pages will tell you all you need to know about the nutrients that will keep you in racing form. We'll start with the most important vitamins and minerals.

VITAMIN C

If you were to take just one supplement a day to help combat stress, it would have to be vitamin C. When we are under stress, vitamin C is used up in fantastic quantities. Indeed, the adrenal glands are the only storehouse in the body for this otherwise unstored, water-soluble vitamin. Humans are one of only seven species in the world which, due to an evolutionary quirk, do not manufacture vitamin C in their bodies. The others are primates, the guinea pig, the Asian red-vented bulbul bird, the Indian fruit-eating bat, the rainbow trout and the Coho salmon.

All other animals increase their vitamin C production when they are under stress. For example, a goat, which normally produces the equivalent of 33mg of vitamin C per kilogramme of body weight a day, will manage to push this up to 190mg when under stress, an increase of more than 500 per cent. Scientists have discovered this fact by carrying out experiments to measure the levels of vitamin C in animals that have just been captured, or which are sick or recovering from surgery, and comparing them to normal levels. It is presumed that humans once had the ability to make vitamin C, but lost it. This is probably because throughout our evolution, our diet included plenty of fruit and vegetables, ensuring that we got all the vitamin C we needed. However, in the period since those remote times, diet changed and the proportion of fruit and vegetables decreased.

VITAMIN C

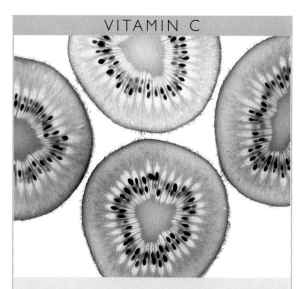

■ Vitamin C is a key component in the manufacture of collagen, which glues our cells together. When the cells of the skin and mucous membranes are not stuck together well, viruses and bacteria are able to breach these protective barriers more easily, resulting in cold sores, colds and flu. The integrity of skin and mucous membranes is important for avoiding eczema and asthma, and repairing wounds.

■ It is a major player in the immune system, necessary for white blood cell manufacture, as well as being antiviral and antibacterial. If there is not sufficient vitamin C available to ensure that enough immune cells are produced to fight diseases, we are open to a whole host of possible illnesses.

■ As if this were not enough, vitamin C is also used for energy production (the citric acid cycle) in every single cell in our body. If these needs are not sufficiently met you can imagine the impact.

■ If the available vitamin C is diverted to support the adrenal glands when we are stressed, all these systems can go wrong.

The importance of vitamin C becomes self-evident when you think about the impact of stress on various systems of the body. Increased stress can be responsible for all sorts of ailments that are improved by vitamin C, such as cold sores, slow healing of wounds, asthma, eczema and lowered immunity to cold and flu viruses.

VITAMIN C SUPPLEMENTS

Extrapolating the figures available for other mammals seems to indicate that, ideally, humans need between 500mg and 5g of vitamin C a day. It is probably wise to take at least 500mg to 1g as a preventive daily dose, increasing this to 3g daily, or more, when ill or under severe stress. It is best to divide the dose, taking it two or three times throughout the day. The least acidic forms of vitamin C, which are gentle on the stomach, are magnesium ascorbate, potassium ascorbate and calcium ascorbate. Other good types to use are Ester-C, or any vitamin C that comes complete with bioflavanoids, which help its use in the body. There is a slight chance of loose bowel movements if you take too much vitamin C (if this happens, just cut back the dose), however it is not in the least harmful and the levels just described are unlikely to cause a problem. In experiments on rats (more stressed rats!) it has been discovered that mega-doses of vitamin C (equivalent to 10g a day for humans) cut the indicators of physical and emotional stress, improved immunity profiles, and actually lowered levels of adrenaline in the blood.

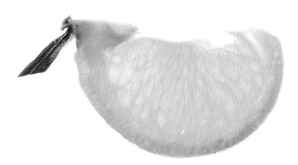

JUICES

Fresh juices are a powerhouse of stress-busting nutrients. Invest in the type of juicer that can handle root vegetables and hard fruit. Your imagination is the only limit for the delicious juices you can create. Some of the vegetables may sound unlikely candidates, for example potatoes, parsnips or cabbage, but try mixing them with a base of carrot or apple juice and taste how great they are. Try some of the following ideas:

For lots of vitamin C
All citrus fruit, strawberries, blackcurrants, blackberries, kiwi fruit, guava, papaya, cabbage, sweet peppers, cauliflower, beansprouts, broccoli, tomatoes, raw potatoes, radishes, parsley.

For high zinc content
Cauliflower, lettuce, berries, cucumber, watermelon with the seeds left in. You can also add in nut milk and/or a spoonful of wheatgerm.

For plenty of magnesium
Green leafy vegetables, broccoli, cabbage, watercress, spinach, kale, spring greens, wheatgrass, grapefruit, carrots, tomatoes. You can also add nut milk (see recipe, right) to the drink.

For good sources of B-vitamins
Green leafy vegetables, apricots, avocado, carrots, bananas, pumpkin, bamboo shoots, parsnip, beetroot, mushrooms. You can blend in banana, avocado, a spoonful of brewer's yeast, yoghurt or half a teaspoon of molasses (molasses has a strong and very sweet, taste).

Foods that are rich in vitamin C include citrus fruit, kiwi fruit, cantaloupe melon, strawberries, peppers, beansprouts, cabbage, broccoli, potatoes, sweet potatoes, rosehip tea, and most other fruits and green leafy vegetables. Vitamin C content is easily destroyed by heating, cooking and storage, so eat lots of fresh fruit, salads and crunchy crudités.

To make nut milk
Take 150g (5oz/1 cup) of nuts (skinned almonds, cashews, or hazelnuts). Put in a blender with 250ml (8fl oz/1 cup) of water and blend at high speed to make a thick cream. Slowly add in more water to achieve the consistency you want – most nut milks use a total of 600ml (1pt/2½ cups) of water to 150g (5oz/1 cup) of nuts. Pass the mixture through a fine sieve. If your nut milk leaves much residue in the sieve, you have not blended it for long enough. To skin almonds, pour boiling water over them and leave for a couple of minutes. Then "pop" the almonds out of their skins. The milk will keep in a fridge for two or three days, and it can be added to a variety of sweet or savoury dishes.

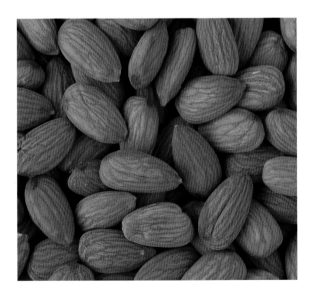

HEALTHY SNACKS TO KEEP IN THE FRIDGE

"Fridge grazing" is an occupational hazard if you are at home. How many times do you go into the kitchen, open the fridge and stare at the contents? As your hand hovers over the salami or cheese, could you make a better choice? Yes, you can. Here are some foods to keep in your fridge or larder for instant snacks, treats or light meals:

■ A selection from the deli counter: houmous, guacamole, salsa, three-bean salad, mushroom paté, tzatziki, mackerel paté. Enjoy any of these with pre-cut vegetable sticks, toasted wholemeal mini-pitta breads or 100 per cent rye crackers.

■ Quartered fruit with cottage cheese. It takes ten seconds to quarter an apple, peach or pear and arrange it on a plate with cottage cheese.

■ Whole celery sticks stuffed with low-fat cream cheese and sprinkled with paprika.

■ Half an avocado with a squeeze of lemon and ground pepper, or stuffed with prawns tossed in plain yoghurt, with chopped herbs.

■ Mashed banana, sprinkled with cinnamon, piled on top of toasted rye bread.

■ Live yoghurt topped with chopped dried fruit, fresh nuts and seeds. For ease you could use trail mix, or stir in some crunchy muesli.

■ Keep a stack of buckwheat pancakes (blinis) in the freezer, separated from each other by greaseproof paper, and pop one in a toaster when you feel peckish. Top with almond butter, apple sauce or slices of kiwi fruit.

■ Wrap strips of cold cuts (chicken, turkey, ham) around dried apricots or prunes and arrange on a plate with carrot and sweet pepper sticks.

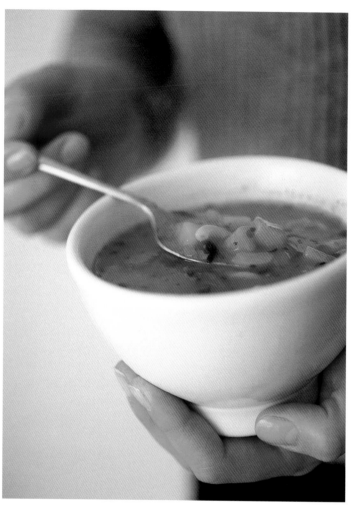

Tasty and tempting, soups are quick and delicious, hot or cold.

■ Soups make an excellent quick light meal or snack – and some are great cold as well as hot. There is a good selection of fresh soups available in the chilled food sections of most supermarkets, but it is easy to make your own, and freshly-made soup can be packed with nutritious ingredients.

■ Make extra amounts of main meals to eat as cold snacks the next day. It is far better to graze on a little leftover stew or cold salmon, rather than to raid the cookie jar.

B-VITAMINS

If you are stressed, tired and anxious, your body is likely to be using more B-vitamins than it would if you were relaxed. It is also quite possible that, to get yourself through difficult times, you will give in to the temptation of sweets, alcohol, coffee and other stimulants. These all deplete B-vitamins, as do certain medications, especially the contraceptive pill, antibiotics and steroids.

The B-vitamins are a family of vitamins labelled by the numbers 1 to 17, which also includes folic acid, choline, biotin and PABA (as well as others). B-vitamins are not stored in the body because they are water-soluble, and so they must be obtained daily from the diet. They are involved in protecting the nervous system, and in metabolizing food to produce energy. Vitamin B5, also called pantothenic acid, is particularly important for the production of adrenal hormones, and a lack of it can bring about adrenal fatigue. Vitamin B6 deficiency has been shown to be a significant factor in the onset of depression, a lack of energy, and

confused mood states. This vitamin is involved in making serotonin, and low levels of this brain chemical are associated with these problems.

The energy cycle, which takes place in each and every cell, is dependent upon B-vitamins. Vitamins B1, B2, B3 and B5 are involved in producing energy from carbohydrates and fats, while B6, B12 and folic acid are important in the conversion of proteins into energy. One of the main signs of a deficiency in B-vitamins is a reduction in energy levels – and of course, when we do not have enough energy, we are less likely to handle stress well.

In general, deficiency of B-vitamins can be recognized by fatigue, depression, insomnia, anxiety, hormonal upsets and skin problems. If you have cracked lips, or cracking at the corner of the mouth, then this is a strong indicator of deficiency. Reducing use of stimulants and increasing intake of vitamin B-rich foods will bring greater relaxation, improved sleep, and help to relieve depression.

B-COMPLEX SUPPLEMENTS

It is always best to take B-vitamins in the form of a complex, because they work best in unison. If you think that you need a "therapeutic" dose of a particular B-vitamin, for instance B5 to help adrenal activity, it is fine to take the isolated vitamin, but best to take a B-complex alongside it. Vitamin B2 is one constituent of a B-complex tablet, and will turn your urine bright yellow. This can be alarming if you are not expecting it, but it does not have any ill-

effects. Another possible reaction is a flushing sensation, a little like a hot sweat, which may be experienced after taking more than 100mg of vitamin B3, also called niacin. This is not in any way harmful, and in fact has certain benefits. B-vitamins are water-soluble and therefore reasonably non-toxic. Most people will benefit from taking a supplement containing 25–100mg of the majority of the B-vitamins.

FOOD SOURCES OF B-VITAMINS

wholegrains

yeast extract

green leafy vegetables

yoghurt

liver

figs

dates

eggs

molasses

nuts

chicken

tuna

sardines

mackerel

cantaloupe melon

cabbage

milk

kale

pumpkin

beans

avocado

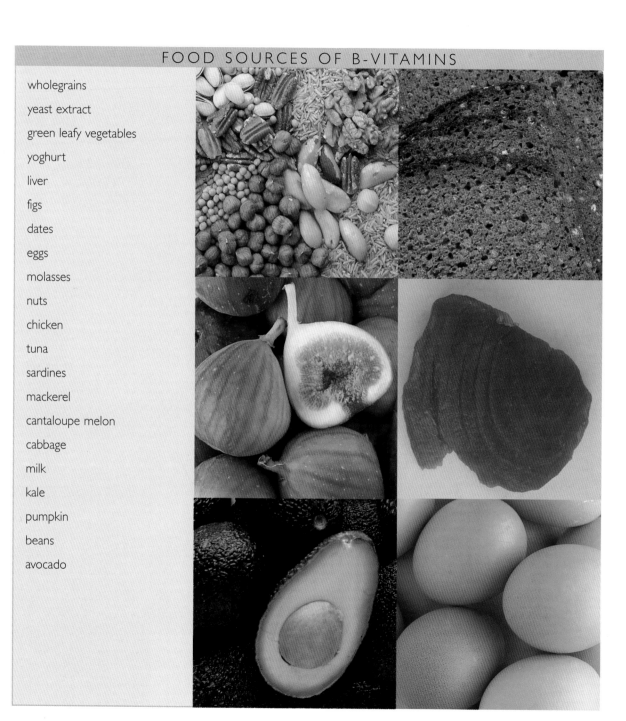

SMOOTHIES

Smoothies are delicious, healthy drinks, made out of soft fruit, which can be whizzed up in five minutes in a high-speed blender. To add to the flavour and nutrient content of your smoothies, you can also include other ingredients. You can make smoothies lighter and fresher tasting by dropping in a handful of ice cubes, or blend in some milk or yoghurt to ensure a thick, luscious creation. You can freeze either of these to make an ice-cream dessert. A smoothie is quite filling, so it makes a good, nourishing substitute for breakfast when you are in a hurry.

Here are some suggestions for making mouthwatering, health-enhancing smoothies:

■ The basic ingredients are the soft fruit of your choice, with milk or water. Skimmed milk, soya milk, coconut milk, rice milk or oat milk may be used instead, and will give your smoothie a rich creamy texture that is totally sin-free. The availability of soft fruit will largely be governed by the season, but include red berries whenever possible because they contain vitamin C and other antioxidants called proanthocyanins. Other suitable candidates are ripe pears, kiwi fruit, papaya, grapes, peaches, plums, banana, mango, melon or watermelon – let your imagination run wild.

■ The inclusion of frozen banana, or ice cubes, will chill a smoothie instantly and give it a refreshing quality. To freeze bananas, peel them and pack them into a rigid container. Put in the freezer and take them out as needed. There is no need to defrost them – blend straight into the smoothie.

■ Live yoghurt (look for "bio" yoghurt) is a good source of beneficial bacteria for the gut.

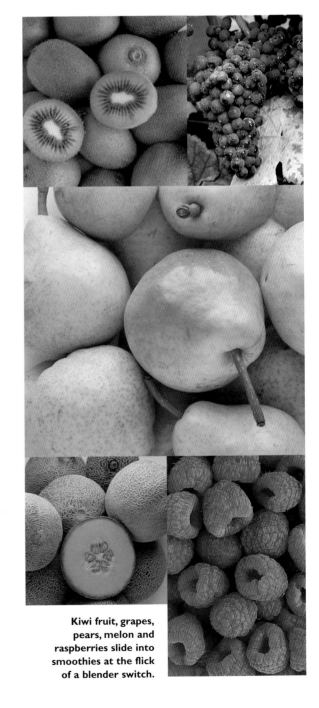

Kiwi fruit, grapes, pears, melon and raspberries slide into smoothies at the flick of a blender switch.

Smoothies make fast, nutritious snacks or meal substitutes.

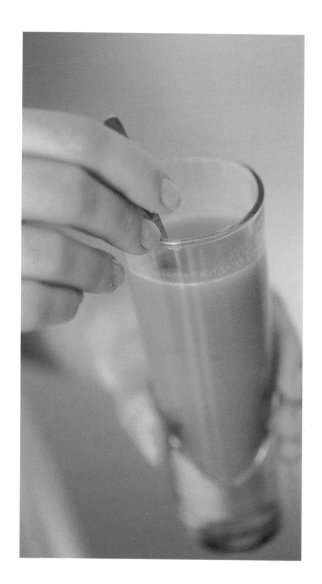

■ Tofu is great for helping to balance female hormones. The "silken" texture type is best, but any will do.

■ You can boost the fibre, mineral and healthy fat content of a smoothie by including seeds. Grind flax, pumpkin, hemp, sunflower or sesame seeds in a clean coffee grinder and add them to the mixture in the blender.

■ A teaspoonful or two of "green food powder" containing some of the following ingredients: chlorella, spirulina, green wheat powder, alfalfa, blue-green algae, seaweeds, green barley or others.

■ A spoonful of any of the following will bring benefits: brewer's yeast contains loads of B-vitamins, wheatgerm is rich in B-vitamins, zinc and magnesium, blackstrap molasses is full of calcium as well as being an excellent source of most other minerals.

■ You can add in any powdered or liquid supplements, as well as the contents of vitamin or mineral capsules. Some people find that the taste of B-vitamins is rather too strong for this. It is not a good idea to include digestive aids that contain hydrochloric acid. Vitamin C powder, aloe vera juice, and many other herbal supplements are suitable candidates.

Things turn out best for the people who make
the best out of the way things turn out.

ART LINKLETTER

MAGNESIUM

This important mineral is named after the Greek city of Magnesia, where large reserves of magnesium carbonate were found. Magnesium is the "life blood" of plants. The chlorophyll molecule, which is responsible for the green colouring of plants, is identical to haemoglobin, the oxygen-carrying factor in our blood, in every respect except one. Chlorophyll uses magnesium, whereas haemoglobin uses iron. Chlorophyll converts sunlight into stored energy in the plant, so when we eat green plants, we are consuming that energy store.

Magnesium is involved in 300 separate functions, that we know of, in the body. It is used during the stress reaction, so long-term stress will push up the requirement for magnesium, which means that the other body processes dependent on it are not adequately supported.

Magnesium is vital for the nervous system and it is particularly effective at dealing with cramp of any sort, from eyelid fluttering to leg cramps which can, in most cases, be viewed as a sign of magnesium deficiency. Other symptoms of deficiency include insomnia, nervousness, depression, high blood pressure, constipation, breast tenderness and water retention. Magnesium works together with vitamins B1 and B6, and is involved in protein synthesis. It is required for the production of certain hormones, making it very useful for the treatment of premenstrual problems.

This magical mineral is available in a wide range of wholefoods, but modern convenience foods, especially milled grains, are sadly stripped of it. Drinking alcohol depletes our magnesium reserves, and also reduces our absorption of magnesium from food. Supplementing with magnesium can help to reduce the risk of adrenal exhaustion caused by long-term stress.

CALCIUM

Magnesium can almost be viewed as as the forgotten mineral. Calcium is given a much wider press and is one of the first minerals that most people think of when contemplating improving their health. And yet calcium is not able to operate properly without the presence of magnesium. Calcium works with magnesium for nerve

Don't be afraid of long silences – communication is about more than words.

ANON

FOOD SOURCES OF MAGNESIUM

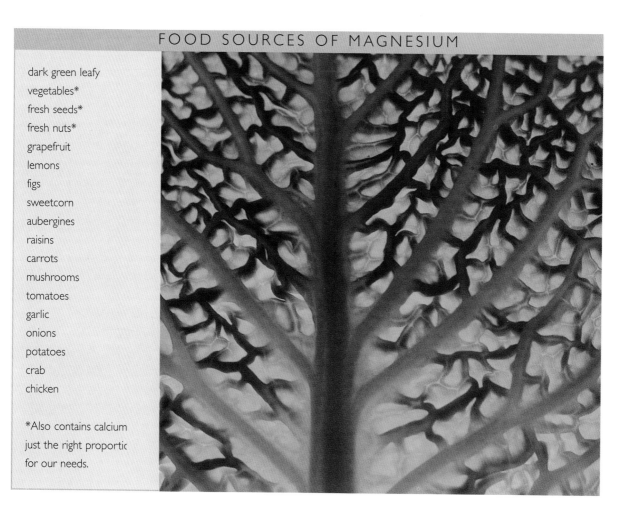

dark green leafy
vegetables*

fresh seeds*

fresh nuts*

grapefruit

lemons

figs

sweetcorn

aubergines

raisins

carrots

mushrooms

tomatoes

garlic

onions

potatoes

crab

chicken

*Also contains calcium
just the right proportic
for our needs.

function, so it is important to maintain the balance between the two minerals for successful stress management.

MAGNESIUM SUPPLEMENTS

We need a dietary ratio of two parts calcium to one part magnesium, but because we get calcium fairly readily from dairy foods, a ratio of one part magnesium to one part calcium is generally suggested for supplementation – for instance 400mg of magnesium to 400mg of calcium. If, however, you have been deficient in magnesium for a while, and are experiencing symptoms such as cramps, it may be helpful to take a ratio of two parts magnesium to one part calcium instead (for example, 600mg magnesium to 300mg of calcium), for three to six months. You can then switch to the "normal" ratio.

ZINC

Zinc is a trace mineral, which we need in minute quantities. However, it is absolutely critical for the growth and repair of all body tissues. Protein foods are broken down, absorbed and go to produce body tissues, nerve chemicals, enzymes and hormones. Zinc is needed for every single stage of protein metabolism: the health benefits of ensuring that you have sufficient zinc in your diet are wide ranging. Women often find that pregnancy leaves them very deficient in zinc, and baby boys take up more zinc than baby girls! Zinc is needed to produce adrenal hormones, and so when protecting yourself from the impact of stress, it is very important to keep zinc at optimal levels. Skin may show signs of damage when we are under stress, and this may be partly due to a lack of zinc, because it is vital for skin building and repair.

Our diet frequently does not contain enough zinc, and statistics show that 31 per cent of women and men do not get the minimum recommended levels suggested. Unfortunately, intensive farming methods have resulted in foods becoming severely depleted in zinc during the last 50 years, and because zinc is not considered essential for optimal plant growth, it is not added into the soil.

Zinc also distinguishes itself by being absolutely necessary for mental function, and low levels are linked to depression, fatigue and loss of libido. Zinc is stored in different tissues in the body, but for men it is most concentrated in their prostate gland and semen, which is an indication of its importance for male sexual function. Zinc is also needed for female sex hormones. The aphrodisiac property of oysters is thought to be linked to their extremely high zinc levels – if you don't like oysters, then a supplement may have to do!

ZINC SUPPLEMENTS

People who are on the go all the time often find it hard to get enough zinc in their diets and may prefer to take a zinc supplement. A maximum safe level is up to 25mg; most high-dose multiple supplements contain around 10mg. If you are going to take a high dose over a long time, then it would be wise to use a supplement that has a little copper in it – 1mg for every 10mg zinc. Zinc is a very safe mineral to supplement at these levels, however some people find that it makes them feel a little nauseous, in which case they should ensure that it is taken with a meal, try a different brand, or failing that, give it up.

SIGNS OF ZINC DEFICIENCY

- White marks on more than two nails
- Paler skin than normal
- Stretch-marks
- Poor sense of taste (may use a lot of salt)
- Poor sense of smell

- Loss of appetite
- Low fertility
- Frequent infections
- A tendency to depression
- Loss of libido

FOOD SOURCES OF ZINC

seeds

nuts

lean meat

seafood

lentils

wholewheat pasta

muesli

oysters

popcorn

wholemeal bread

beans

leafy green vegetables

eggs

hard cheeses

wholegrains

yoghurt

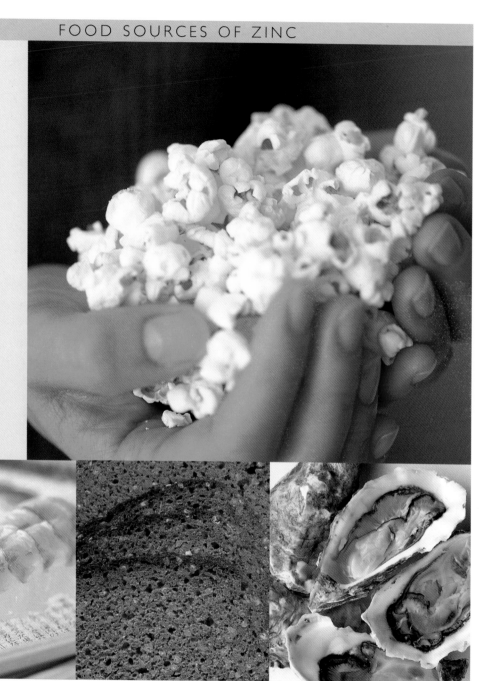

Water

Our bodies are 70 per cent water; even our seemingly dry bones are 10 per cent water. Water is used for every function in the body: it maintains homeostasis, or balance, in the cells; it is the solvent in which minerals and other matter are carried around the body; it is used for every enzyme process that governs the nerve chemicals, and therefore every thought and action, every chemical process and therefore every function, in the body. So it goes without saying that we need to drink a lot of it. Dehydration can be responsible for creaking and stiff joints, constipation, dry skin conditions, fatigue, hunger, headaches, dizziness, lung and urinary infections.

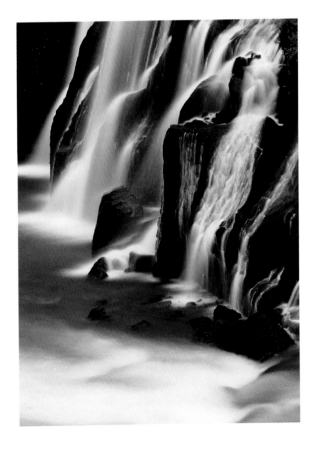

If you suspect that you not drink enough water (40 per cent of people do not), try this little experiment. Take an empty bottle that holds two litres (3½ pints/10 cups) – the amount of water we need to drink daily – and as you prepare each cup of tea or coffee during the day, pour an equivalent amount of water into the bottle. You will discover that you easily consume this amount of liquid – all you need to do is to make a switch from one type of drink to another. As well as drinking more water, replace tea and coffee, at least partially, with herb or fruit teas, or coffee substitutes made with dandelion, chicory, barley or rye. Give up at least a part of your alcohol intake in favour of diluted fruit juices, sparkling water with ice and a slice of lemon, or herbal cocktail drinks readily available from healthfood stores. Of course, water also has many therapeutic uses: we bathe in it, use it for massage, and suspend aromatic oils in it. Water really has magical properties.

Water is crucial to health – we need to drink eight glasses daily for body systems to operate efficiently.

TOP FIVE HYDRATION TREATMENTS

1 Every day, drink between six and eight large glasses of water with a squeeze of lemon and a sprig of mint.

2 Make sure that you eat five pieces of really juicy fruit every day.

3 Herbal and fruit teas make a refreshing change to caffeine-laden tea and coffee. Make a jug of iced herbal tea with mint leaves, orange slices and a little honey – with such a visual treat you will never feel deprived of your usual brew.

4 Next time you feel peckish, drink a glass of water. You may be mistaking hunger pangs for thirst signals.

5 Avoid dehydrating drinks. The worst are alcohol, coffee, tea and colas.

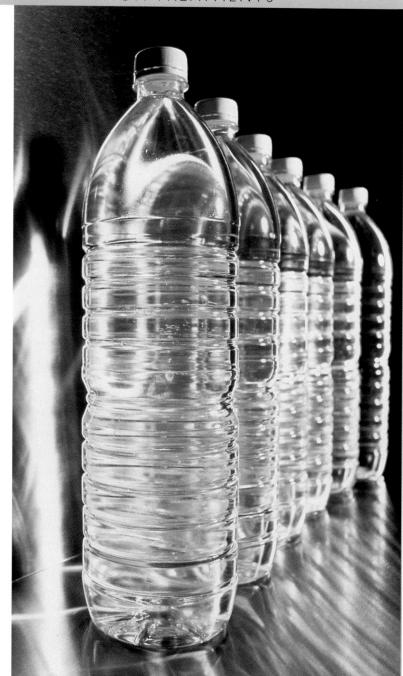

WATER THERAPIES

In 1880, Dr William Winternitz, an Austrian physician, discovered that water acts on the nerve points (reflex or pressure points) on the skin, in a similar way to acupuncture or acupressure. Water comes in the form of ice, liquid and steam, and each has various uses. Ice packs help to relieve pain, warm water compresses ease muscle tension, and steam is a potent carrier of healing scents – extremely therapeutic in a steam room.

Alternate hot and cold hand bath

This is wonderful for stimulating the reflex points in your hands, because all the Chinese energy meridians used in acupuncture begin or end in the hands. Fill two containers, one with very hot water (as hot as you can stand, but do not burn yourself), and one with very cold water. Plunge your hands in the hot water for three minutes, and then into the cold water for half a minute. Repeat three times, and always end with the cold water to restore muscle tone.

Cold water treading

This is an invigorating treatment, which encourages a feeling of euphoria. Use it for nervousness, insomnia, exhaustion, weakness, aching feet, chilblains and catarrhal nose or throat conditions. As well as all these, it is a useful preventive therapy, which helps to build the immune response. Stand in a bathtub filled with cold water up to the level of your ankles. March on the spot for up to five minutes. Hold on to a handrail or use a non-slip rubber mat in the bath for safety. Do not do this if you have rheumatism, sciatica or inflamed pelvic conditions.

Sitz bath

This is one of the oldest naturopathic treatments, where you sit in a bath containing hot water, with your feet in another bath containing cold water, and vice versa. Altering the temperature of one area of the body can have profound effects on the rest of the body. To create this energizing and tonic effect for yourself, fill the bath with a few inches of hot water and sit in it (take care not to burn yourself). After a few minutes, change to a cold bath. Repeat the process.

Jet spray

One of the nicest treatments available at health spas is a high-powered spray massage treatment. This is easy to replicate at home if you have a garden, a garden hosepipe fitted with a high-pressure nozzle, fine weather, a willing and responsible friend, and a sense of humour. Put on your swimming costume, and ask your friend to turn the hose on you, working from your feet up towards your shoulders. By starting with the feet you can get used to the coldness of the water, then the massage should be moved slowly in the direction of your heart. At no time should the water jet be used near the head. This treatment is amazingly invigorating and great fun.

SURROUND YOURSELF WITH SCENT

In Roman times, the communal baths were a central part of life, where people could socialize and indulge in soothing therapies such as steam baths, ice rubs, or massage with warm olive oil. The use of oils and essential oils for massage and other therapies has continued through the centuries. Certain essential oils have a beneficial effect on emotions and moods, the ability to manage stress, and help to ensure a peaceful night's rest. They can help to keep spirits high in the face of adversity and encourage the release of negative emotions. You can use them in a number of ways:

Bath

Run a warm bath and add three to six drops of essential oils. You can mix several oils together to suit your mood, but do not be tempted to use a total of more than six drops.

Massage

Put 50ml (2fl oz) of a base oil such as almond, walnut, sunflower seed, apricot kernel or peach kernel into a clean bottle. Add 20 drops of your chosen essential oil or oils, and shake well. Use the blend to gently massage the skin. Do not apply to areas of broken skin. This amount is sufficient for several treatments.

Steam inhalation

Add two to four drops of your chosen essential oil to a bowl containing 600ml (1pt/2½ cups) of boiling water. Sit down and place the bowl in front of you, put a towel over your head and the bowl, and inhale the vapours. Be careful not to get too close to the boiling water.

Room scent

Buy an essential oil burner or vaporizer to spread therapeutic vapours round your room. It has a saucer into which you put a little water and a couple of drops of your chosen oil, and a candle burns underneath it. Electrically operated vaporizers are also available.

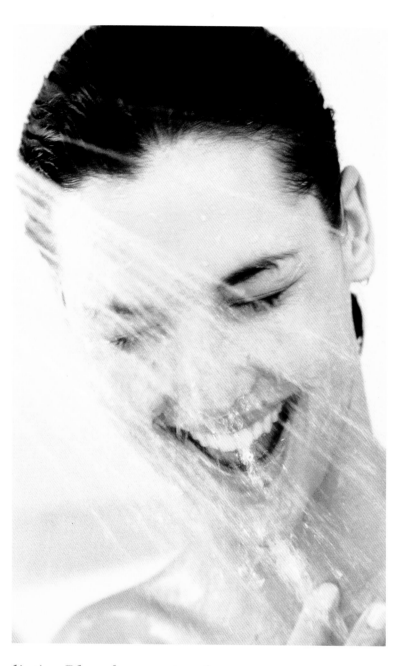

The jet spray uses a blast of cold water to provide a massage treatment that will invigorate the whole body.

Be realistic. Plan for a miracle.

BHAGWAN SHREE RAJNEESH

The essential guide to herbal stress-busters

Herbs are potent health modulators and can deal with symptoms of stress effectively. Some, such as chamomile, are known to be particularly safe. However, many herbs must not be taken during pregnancy. If you are pregnant, or on any medication, get professional advice from a herbalist about contra-indications, before taking any herbs.

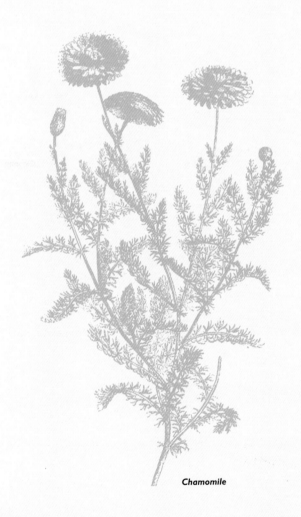

Chamomile

DAMIANA

This herb not only energizes the nervous system and acts as an antidepressant, but can also give your sex life a boost! It stimulates the reproductive system and is an aphrodisiac.

Tea: 1 tsp herb in a cup of boiling water. Leave to infuse for 15 minutes. You may find that one cup three times a day is sufficient.

Capsules: Take a 300mg capsule three times a day.

Liquid extract: ½–1 tsp in water three times daily.

BORAGE

A reviving herb that stimulates the adrenal glands. Good for chronic stress, during steroid treatment, and for menopausal problems. Add it to drinks, or include young leaves in salads. Older leaves can be eaten as a vegetable. The seeds are a good source of the essential fatty acid GLA.

Tea: 1 tsp herb in a cup of boiling water. Infuse for 15 minutes.

Liquid extract: ½–1 tsp in water three times daily.

CHAMOMILE

Dissipates tension without the side-effect of sedation. Chamomile can help when everything seems unbearable, lifting depression and relieving nausea caused by emotional

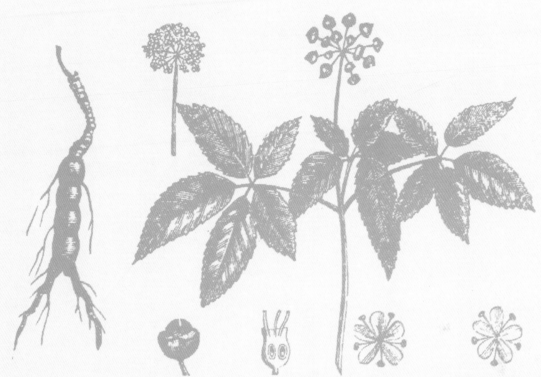

Ginseng

upsets. German chamomile (wild chamomile) is the most potent; Roman chamomile is less bitter. Both chamomiles are diuretic, which makes them particularly useful for easing premenstrual water retention. They also relieve premenstrual tension.

Tea: 1 tsp herb in a cup of boiling water. Infuse for ten minutes.

VERVAIN

Vervain relaxes muscles that are affected by stress and tension. It is used to treat nervous breakdowns, depression and chronic fatigue.

Tea: 1–2 tsp dried herb per cup of boiling water. Infuse for 15 minutes. One cup three times daily.

Capsules: 1–4g dried herb three times a day.

GINSENG, KOREAN

In Chinese medicine, this is the number one herb for bolstering the biochemical reaction to stress. You can obtain it as dried root, or in capsules, powders and teas.

High-quality crude ginseng root: 1–2g, one to three times a day.

Standardized extract (five per cent ginsenosides): 100mg, one to three times a day.

GINSENG, SIBERIAN

This herb only came to the attention of Western herbalists in the last century, but since then it has been studied extensively, particularly for its anti-stress properties.

Dried root: 2–4g, three times daily. Usually taken for between one week and one month (it is best not to exceed this length of time). Do not take with coffee, because the overall effect will be too stimulating; in cases of hyperactivity it should also be avoided.

OATS

Oats have a higher amount of iron and zinc than any other grain, and exert a calming effect on the nervous system. You are better off having a bowl of porridge, some oatcakes or an oatmeal-based drink to calm your nerves than many other options. A hyperactive child would benefit from having porridge for breakfast. Avoid taking passion flower at the same time as oats, but a cup of valerian tea, on the other hand, complements the properties of oats.

Oatmeal: Take as porridge, stirred into soups or used as topping, or as a hot oatmeal drink.

Liquid extract: 1–2ml in water three times daily. Avoid in cases of gluten sensitivity.

LADY'S SLIPPER

This herb is also known as nerve root, because it calms the nerves and alleviates nervousness and anxiety. The sedative properties of Lady's slipper were recognized by the Native Americans. Today it is used to treat irritability, premenstrual tension, depression, weepiness, and insomnia due to worry.

Root powder: 2–4g, three times daily.

Liquid extract: ½–1 tsp in water three times daily.

Tea: 1 tsp dried herb per cup of water. Boil the herb in the water for a couple of minutes, then leave to infuse for a further 15 minutes.

LAVENDER

A wonderfully relaxing herb. Lavender tea can be used to relieve stress at the end of a tough day, to lift mild depression, and to speed recovery from tension headaches

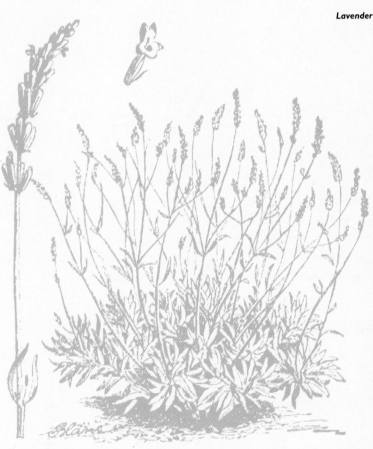

Lavender

and migraines. A few drops of essential oil can added to the bath to soothe aching muscles, or used in a vaporizer to instil a feeling of calmness.

Tea: A third of a teaspoonful of dried lavender per cup of water. Drink three times daily.

Capsules: 500mg, three times daily.

ROSE

Both the petals and rosehips of the rose can be made into a tea. Rosehip tea (easily available from healthfood stores) is rich in vitamin C. Rose petal tea can be made by steeping petals in boiling water. They both have an uplifting effect on the nervous system. Rose tea reduces tension and anxiety, helps to relieve depression, dispels mental fatigue and smooths away irritability. When gathering petals or hips yourself, ensure that the plant has not been sprayed with chemicals. Rosewater, available from the chemist, can be used to relieve tired and sore eyes.

Tea: 20–30 petals infused in boiling water for 10 minutes.

KAVA KAVA

For hundreds of years, South Pacific islanders have made a tea from kava kava to induce a state of relaxation and tranquillity. Scientific investigation has proved that it has an anti-anxiolytic (anxiety-reducing) and calming effect on the nerves, and also on migraines and premenstrual cramps. These qualities have given rise to its nickname of the "herbal Valium". It also has muscle relaxant and analgesic properties.

Capsules: 150mg of standardized root extract three times daily.

Liquid extract: ½–1 tsp in water three times daily. Taking more than the recommended dose may cause dry skin and a rash, which disappear when the use of the herb is discontinued.

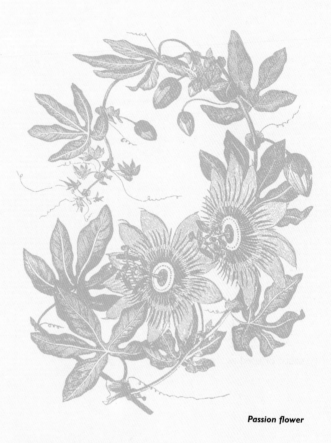

Passion flower

PASSION FLOWER

A great general relaxant, which calms an overactive brain and pounding heart, and is particularly good for relieving insomnia. It is actually a mild sedative: the active compound, chrysin, works by inhibiting a substance called gamma-aminobutyric acid (GABA) in the brain. Other "hypnotic" agents such as kava kava and valerian work in the same way.

Tea: ½ tsp herb in a cup of boiling water, leave to infuse for 15 minutes. Drink before going to bed if you are having trouble sleeping. Do not drink passion flower tea with a meal that includes oats.

Capsules: ½–1g, three times daily.

Liquid extract: 1–2ml, three times daily in water.

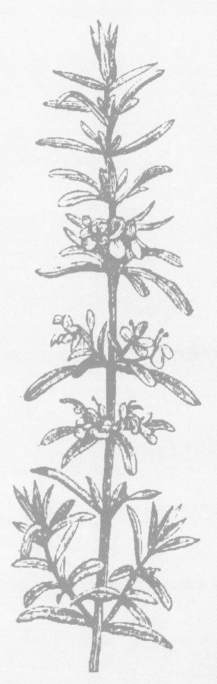

Rosemary

ROSEMARY

Excellent for treating migraines, particularly if brought on by stress, also good for headaches caused by high blood pressure. Rosemary's sedative action makes it useful as a substitute for mild tranquillizers. It is beneficial for those with chronic fatigue.

Tea: ½–1 tsp of rosemary in a cup of boiling water, leave to infuse for 15 minutes. (Cover the cup with a saucer to stop the essential oils from escaping.)

Capsules: 1–4g, three times a day.

Liquid extract: 30–60 drops in water three times a day.

LIQUORICE ROOT

This is not the same as liquorice confectionery! The root affects the part of the adrenal glands concerned with potassium and sodium balance, and reduces stress damage to the adrenal cortex. It has similar anti-inflammatory effects to hydrocortisone and is helpful for dealing with aches and pains. Use the deglycyrrhized version (DGL) to avoid depleting your potassium levels. It can be helpful during the transition phase of reducing steroid medication (but not without your doctor's knowledge). Avoid in cases of high blood pressure, fluid retention, or during pregnancy.

Dried root: 1–4g, three times daily. You can also buy liquorice root sticks, to chew on, from healthfood stores.

ROYAL JELLY

Royal jelly is a concentrated food that worker bees secrete from their salivary glands. The queen bee feeds on it, enabling her to live 30 times longer than other bees. Royal jelly helps us to ward off infections, and also boosts energy and improves the health of skin, hair and nails. It is a great antidote to stress – probably because it contains almost all the B-vitamins and vitamin C. Royal jelly is widely available in capsule form. You can also get it in tiny vials with a miniature straw to suck out the jelly from each one. Delicious!

Capsules: 500mg daily.

SKULLCAP

Skullcap is helpful for treating nervous stress caused by just about any physical or mental excess: workaholics who suffer from mental exhaustion, people with long-term illness, those who over-exercise, and people who feel that life is a constant slog with no let-up. It is also very useful for insomniacs and for soothing any tension in the body such as PMT, shock, and stress-related headaches and migraines.

Tea: ½ tsp of skullcap in a cup of boiling water; infuse for 15 minutes.

Capsules: ½–2g dried herb, three times a day.

ST. JOHN'S WORT

Sometimes known as the "nerve-herb", this is a natural antidepressant suitable for mild to moderate depression, which allows the brain to process pleasurable feelings instead of blocking them. It does this by restoring the communication links between nerve endings, and by raising serotonin levels. St. John's wort does not have the side-effects of

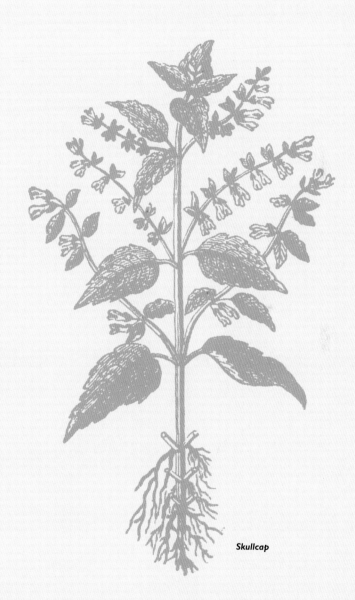

Skullcap

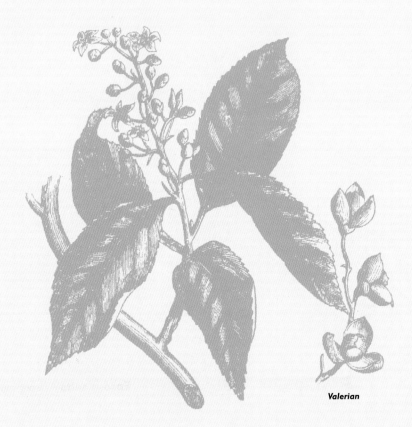

Valerian

antidepressant drugs. Its benefits include the lifting of low moods, improved alertness and enhanced mental performance. It can also eliminate despair, anxiety, insomnia and tension headaches. The sixteenth-century Swiss physician, Paracelsus, said of St. John's wort that "every physician should know that God has blessed the herb with a great, mysterious power, that will protect one from such spirits as cause bewilderment".

Capsules: 1–4g dried root, three times daily. Side-effects are virtually unknown at recommended doses, but may cause photosensitivity, and must not be used with medication or other antidepressants.

VALERIAN ROOT

Valerian is used as a gentle non-addictive tranquillizer, and its ability to calm both body and mind has been known since ancient times. It is used for many of the symptoms of stress, such as insomnia, menstrual pain, muscle cramps, high blood pressure and tension headaches, and it is also useful for decreasing feelings of restlessness in menopausal women.

Tea: Infuse ½ tsp of dried root in a cup of boiling water for 15 minutes. Drink three times a day.

Capsules: Take one 1000mg capsule in the morning and one in the evening.

DONG QUAI

The dried root is used widely for female hormonal problems, such as mood swings, anxiety, depression, weepiness, menopausal symptoms and fatigue, all of which are more likely to be a problem during times of stress. In the East, it is known as the female ginseng (see *ginseng*). Dong quai can directly help stress by lowering high blood pressure and encouraging a restful night's sleep.

Capsules: 2–6g, three times a day.

HERBAL BATHS

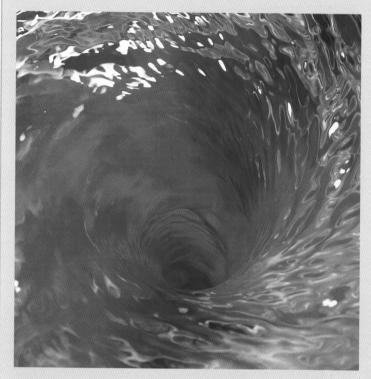

Try adding herbs and other substances from your kitchen cupboards to your bath for a variety of effects. Some herbs soothe, some sedate or stimulate and others just soften the skin and feel nice! End your bath with a vigorous rub-down with a towel.

Apple cider vinegar Helps to combat fatigue and restore the natural acid covering of the skin.

Chamomile flowers or an infusion of chamomile is useful for inflamed skin or skin rashes.

Epsom salts A strong muscle relaxant. Encourages perspiration, which is excellent for detoxification.

Oatmeal Soothes the skin and is great for eczema.

Rosemary Stimulates and increases blood circulation, helping to combat mental fatigue.

Salt Helps to heal and tranquillize. A rub with coarse sea salt before a bath is an excellent exfoliator and is very invigorating. Be careful not to apply salt to broken skin. Sea salt is best.

Good timber does not grow with ease.

The stronger the wind, the stronger the trees.

J. WILLARD MARRIOT

the stress protection plan
overview

Change your life and banish stress for good.
Stress-busting plans to set you on the right track.

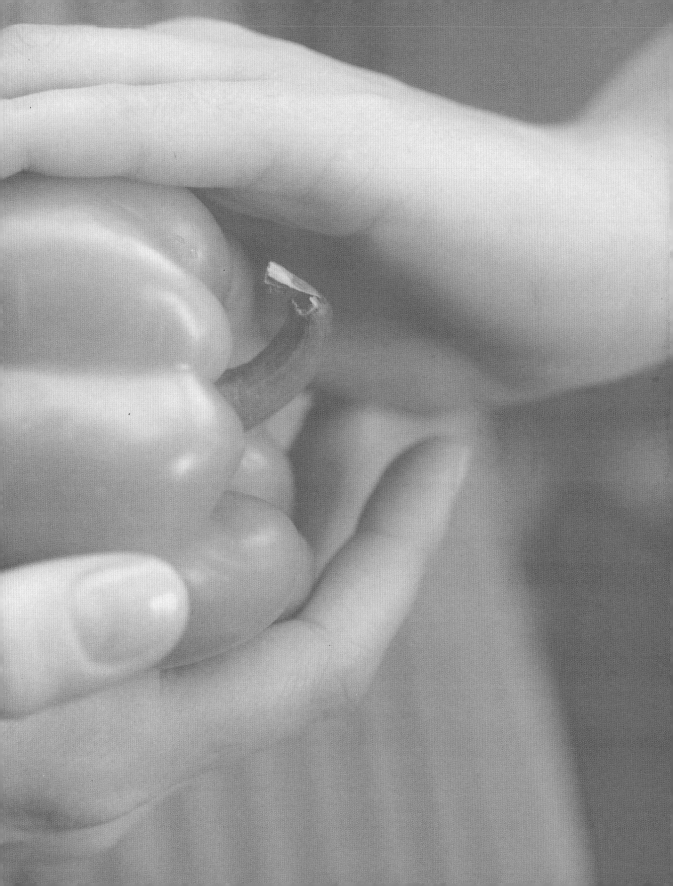

Making changes

Many of us have an overwhelming desire to renew ourselves. You have the potential to do whatever you set your mind to, and now is the time for action. This section of the book shows you how to utilize the theories we have already discussed, in order to realize your true potential.

Taking action is the key to everything. Succeed in creating new habits that stick. A number of stress protection plan options are outlined later in the chapter. There are three weekend plans, for boosting your energy levels, dealing with hectic times, or for detoxifying your body. The one-week plan is suitable for a holiday break, or as a preparation for more significant changes. There is also a one-month plan, which takes a more comprehensive approach.

Beating stress means changing ingrained habits, but all the plans are easy to follow. You gently ease into a new framework of looking after yourself and attending to your own needs. The most difficult aspect of this is usually setting time aside for yourself!

The exercises in this book are all meant to be practised. It is not enough to read about them and to hope that they will somehow permeate your life. Each week, or each month, incorporate one exercise into your life, and it will soon become a habit. Most of the exercises can be adapted to suit your needs.

As you progress through the plans you will relax, feel better about yourself, have more energy, sleep more soundly, and feel refreshed. Your increased vitality can be channelled into exercise and other activities you enjoy. You should find that you become less susceptible to colds and other ailments. Long-standing troubles, such as PMS, headaches, migraines, aching joints, digestive troubles and eczema may begin to vanish. The condition of skin and hair will improve.

BE REALISTIC

Make your goals realistic. Deciding to go and climb Mount Everest tomorrow is unrealistic. However, going for a one-hour walk, to start your exercise regime, is easily achievable. And then maybe one day you will get to climb Everest! You need to marry your potential to a genuine belief in yourself and your abilities. You then need to act. This is crucial for getting results. The fundamental difference between people who succeed at their goals and those who don't is that those who succeed are specific about their goals, while those who fail are often vague. Those who succeed usually take action decisively, while those who don't just talk.

If you have previously succeeded in one of your goals, you have a terrific advantage. You know you can do such a thing. You can retrace the steps that helped you to win, and apply those principles to other areas of your life. If your plans repeatedly fall by the wayside you need to examine ways to break your goals into easy steps and act on them. The following questions will help you identify why previous attempts at change have failed.

WHAT HAS STOPPED YOU IN THE PAST?

Attempting to change lifestyle factors

■ Did you set realistic goals with manageable stepping stones along the way?

■ Were you consistent in your behaviour?

■ Were you doing too many things at the same time?

■ What stood in the way of change? Was it outside forces, or internal conflicts?

Attempting to change eating habits

■ Did you fully take into account potential obstacles such as the demands of your social, work and family life?

■ Did you make too many dietary changes in one go?

■ Did you find sufficient alternative foods and drinks?

■ Did you feel deprived by the changes?

■ Did you feel good about the changes? Did they empower and motivate you? How long did your sense of motivation last? What interrupted these feelings?

TACKLING CHANGE SUCCESSFULLY

Now you have some insight into your behaviour patterns, you can concentrate on making changes that will stick.

■ What are your three most important goals in nutritional or lifestyle areas? (Pick one short-term goal, one medium-term goal, and one long-term goal.)

■ For each goal, make a comprehensive list of every step required to achieve it. This is now your route-map.

■ Have you previously attempted to reach these three goals and failed? What will make you succeed?

■ What are your plans for overcoming the obstacles that will try and trip you up? Can you foresee the obstacles?

■ How will you know when you have attained your goals? It is not enough to say that you want to be stress-free, or to lose weight. You must specify, for example, that you want to be able to sleep well, or to lose 4.5kg (10lb). What are the markers of success for you?

■ What will your rewards be when you succeed?

BACH FLOWER REMEDIES

Flower remedies are homeopathically prepared essences, which are mainly used to address emotional imbalances. They are most effective when carefully matched to the personality of the person taking them. A few drops added to water and taken four times a day can help to lift your spirits, calm your mind and focus your energies. Here are a few remedies that may be appropriate for you.

White Chestnut

For those who cannot put aside problems, and who cannot sleep. For mental tension, worry, teeth grinding, chronic headaches, fatigue and depression.

Impatiens

For impatient people, who are always in a hurry, irritable, hard to please and restless.

Elm

For people who are temporarily overwhelmed, especially by responsibility, though normally capable.

Heather

For self-centred people who weep easily, tend to make mountains out of molehills, and feel self-pity. Also for fear of loneliness.

Olive

For complete physical and mental exhaustion after a long period of strain, where the person is washed out and finds everything an effort.

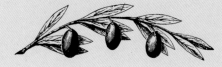

Varying your diet

When we are in a rush and under pressure, a healthy diet is one of the first things to suffer. It is easiest to grab instant meals – pre-packaged, microwaveable, or from the take-away. Even if we cook fresh foods, we often opt for those that are easiest to prepare.

You may think you have a varied diet, but closer scrutiny may reveal that the same ingredients make up a number of dishes or pre-prepared foods, and you are actually dependent on a very small range of "core" foods. For instance, wheat is found in bread, pasta, cakes, biscuits, pastry, pies, cous-cous and cracked wheat (bulgar). It is also mixed into many packaged foods as a bulk filler. Some brands of rye bread, rye crackers, oatcakes or corn cakes also contain significant quantities of wheat, so check the labels before you buy.

THE BENEFITS OF A VARIED DIET ARE TWOFOLD:

● It exposes you to a wider variety of nutrients. If all you eat is wheat bread and wheat pasta, you will only get what wheat has to offer. If, on the other hand, you also eat other grains such as oats, rice, rye, barley, buckwheat, quinoa or millet, you will take in a broader range of nutrients and benefit your health.

● You also reduce the likelihood of developing food allergies and sensitivities, because you are not overexposed to any particular foods. Adverse food reactions can be responsible for, or contribute to, a long list of symptoms including bloating, flatulence, bad breath, loose stools, constipation, irritable bowel syndrome, eczema, psoriasis, palpitations, insomnia, fatigue and arthritis.

BUDGET HEALTHFOODS

A common criticism levelled at healthy foods is that they are expensive, but that is not the case. The foods that really make a hole in a budget are convenience and snack foods. Eating

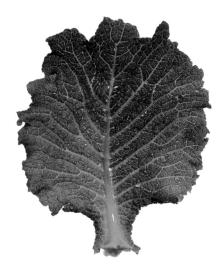

healthily does not depend on exotic foods and beautifully packaged "alternative" foods from the healthfood store. Some of the most beneficial foods are among the cheapest, especially if you buy them in season, and you can store some in your freezer. You may need to invest a little more time in creative cooking, but stress-busting foods that do not cost the earth include:

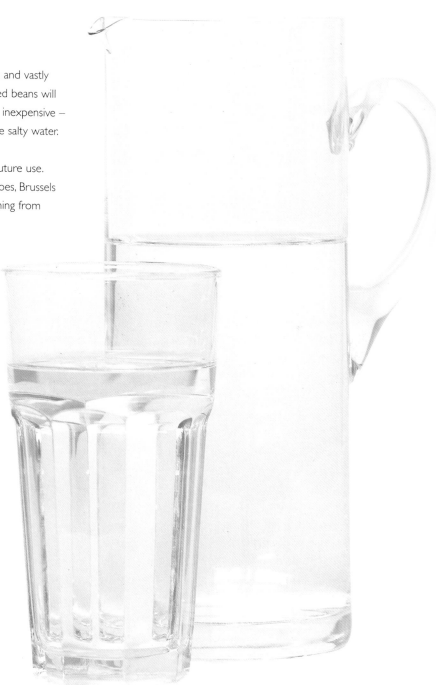

■ Beans and lentils. These are really versatile and vastly underused in Western cuisine. A store of dried beans will last months. Even canned beans are relatively inexpensive – just place them in a colander and rinse off the salty water.

■ Grains such as rice, oats and barley.

■ Fruits in season. These can be frozen for future use.

■ Vegetables such as cabbage, carrots, potatoes, Brussels sprouts and onions can be made into everything from hearty soups to exotic salads.

■ Oily fish, including mackerel, sardines, sprats, herring and pilchards. These are rich in beneficial oils, which fight a number of health conditions.

■ Water. We do not drink enough water. Replace a significant part of your fluid intake with water (filter it if you can) and your health will benefit.

■ Meat is usually the most expensive item in the shopping basket. Use meat in small "Eastern" amounts – such as a little diced chicken or shrimp to go with a stir-fry, or a little meat to bolster a stew.

Our doubts are traitors,
And make us lose the
good we oft might win,
By fearing to attempt.

WILLIAM SHAKESPEARE

Beating addictions

We have already looked at how foods can act in an almost pharmacological way, by directly affecting brain chemicals. We also know that foods affect blood sugar levels, and stimulate adrenaline. The combination of these factors makes many foods highly addictive, especially for people who have a predisposition to dependency.

Ask yourself whether there is any food, or substance, that it would be difficult for you to live without. Most people give answers such as chocolate, bread, cheese, coffee, wine and cigarettes. When the item is avoided for a while, the pay-off in increased energy, reduced stress and improved health can be extraordinary.

A good indication of the strength of the impact foods can have on the body is shown by the symptoms that often occur when they are withdrawn. It is common to have headaches as a result of giving up caffeine, and a few of days of avoiding certain foods can lead to a worsening of problems such as spots, dry skin and bad breath. This is usually followed by a feeling of lightness and energy as the body is freed from the burden of eliminating the toxins normally created by the rogue food. Turn to page 134 for more information about detoxifying your body.

FOOD SENSITIVITIES

Apart from stimulants such as caffeine, sugar and alcohol, foods that most commonly cause sensitivities are wheat and dairy products – which have been shown to have an opium-like effect on the brain. Other foods that often cause sensitivity reactions include grains such as rye, oats, barley and corn, soya foods, potatoes and citrus fruit (especially oranges). If you believe you may be sensitive to a food, it is worth avoiding it for two weeks, and see if you feel any better for doing so. Also, if you get twitchy at the thought of existing for more than a couple of days without the bread, pasta, cheese or sweet foods that you usually enjoy, it indicates that your food addiction may be resulting in health problems. For further information on food addictions see page 22.

How do you go about avoiding particular foods? Do not regard it as deprivation that is being thrust upon you, but focus on what you *can* eat. Plan satisfying meals ahead, and if you are giving up bread and wheat products for a while, experiment with other starchy foods and grains such as potatoes, rice and oats.

Our weakest moments, when we are most likely to revert to previous eating patterns, are usually when we are tired and cannot be bothered to make the effort to stick to our resolutions. This could be breakfast time, mid-afternoon or when we get home in the evening. To avoid succumbing to temptation, work out, in advance, some breakfasts, snacks and meals that will give you an energy boost but will not feed your addictions. Keep the ingredients ready.

**Preventing the
absorption of
minerals is one of
caffeine's crimes.**

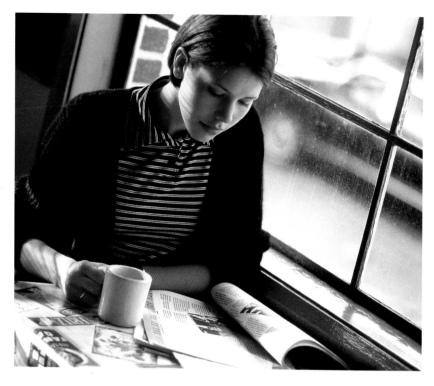

CAFFEINE

Caffeine is a stimulant. It can cause irritability and overstimulate the adrenal glands. In the long term, this can reduce your ability to cope with stress. Even moderate doses of caffeine raise levels of the stress hormones adrenaline and cortisol to levels higher than those produced by the body during a stress reaction. So if you are drinking coffee because you feel stressed, more stress hormones are entering your system than would be triggered solely in response to the stress.

Sources of caffeine include coffee, tea, chocolate, colas, "energy drinks", headache medication, painkillers and the herb guarana. Caffeine prevents the absorption of some essential nutrients, especially zinc (an anti-stress nutrient) and iron (needed for energy).

Strong tea can be as high in caffeine as a cup of coffee. However, if you make weaker tea, two or three cups a day are not detrimental for most people. There are many delicious substitute drinks including dandelion, chicory and barley coffees, herbal and fruit teas and herb drinks. Sometimes the ritual of putting the kettle on to make a hot drink is more important than the drink itself. Many people find that they are just as happy to have a cup of hot water, or hot water and a lemon slice, instead of coffee. The homeopathic remedy Coffea can help to reduce cravings when trying to wean yourself off caffeine.

CHOCOLATE

While chocolate is a source of caffeine, it is also contains a number of other compounds that have profound effects on the body and contribute to the sheer "moreishness" of this seductive food. Chocolate suppresses beta waves in the brain (which are linked to alertness), while raising alpha waves (which increase when people are in a meditative state). It may be that we are unconsciously seeking these calming effects when we reach for chocolate – another reason why chocolate is so addictive. Most chocolate is very high in sugar, so if you are going to buy some, choose 70 per cent cocoa solid chocolate instead, which is lower in sugar. A couple of squares of this is usually sufficient for most chocoholics, and can help to wean you off guzzling large amounts of cheaper brands of chocolate. And you can always console yourself with the fact that good-quality chocolate is also a source of magnesium and antioxidants.

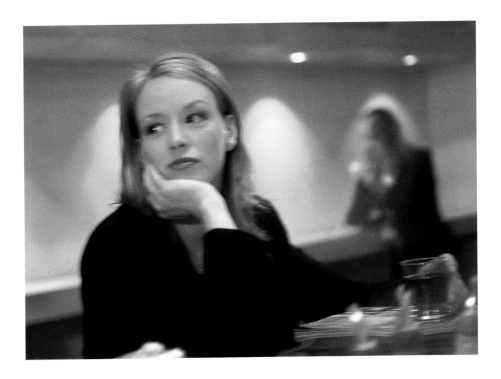

Excessive drinking equals weight gain and depletion of vitamins.

SUGAR

This drug is legal! Sugar impairs the working of the adrenal glands and suppresses the immune system. A massive 80 per cent of the sugar we eat comes from processed foods, and it is an education to read their labels. Look for sucrose, maltose, glucose, lactose and dextrose, which are all sugars. Overcoming the desire for sweet foods goes hand-in-hand with balancing blood sugar levels. For this reason, it is best to concentrate on stress-busting meal choices before you attempt to give up sugary snacks.

Cutting down on sugar can be done gradually, and after about a month your tastebuds will be retrained. Artificial sweeteners are not really a solution because, while they do not trigger blood sugar, they do nothing to retrain your taste for sweetness and are also difficult chemicals for your body to process and eliminate. In moderation, you can use fructose, which is fruit sugar. It is much sweeter than sugar and does not have a severe impact on blood sugar levels. Honey has the same effect as sugar in terms of affecting blood sugar levels, but a little organic raw honey is a healthier option than refined sugar. Raw honey is a source of enzymes and other compounds which have therapeutic benefits with antiseptic properties.

ALCOHOL

Alcohol overstimulates the adrenal glands, and the effect on blood sugar levels and brain chemistry is significant. Though initially a stimulant, the follow-on effect is depressive. Alcohol can trigger a desire to eat more; drinking too much alcohol also provides a lot of calories, which can significantly contribute to weight gain. Excessive drinking depletes vitamins and minerals, and this can make the liver less effective at detoxifying many substances, including the alcohol itself. If you usually drink a little alcohol each day, cut back by drinking only on alternate days. This limits the repetitive "habit-forming" aspect of drinking. Social drinking is very tempting, but you can set yourself rules, such as not drinking at lunchtime, or limiting alcohol to certain days of the week, or using strategies such as drinking a glass of water for each glass of alcohol. You could also volunteer to drive when you go out for the evening, which gives you the perfect excuse to be on the wagon.

BETTER CHOICES

INSTEAD OF	CHOOSE
Coffee	Barley, chicory or dandelion coffee.
Strong tea	Weak tea, green tea, rooibos, luaka tea, ginger tea, mint tea, fruit tea, hot cordial (choose 80 per cent fruit cordial, or make your own using fructose or stevia).
An alcoholic drink	A spicy tomato juice, sparkling water with ice and a slice, herbal drink (for example, Aqualibra or Amé), spritzer (half white wine, half sparkling water – still alcohol but 50 per cent better for you than drinking wine on its own), cordial (choose 80 per cent fruit cordial, or make your own using fructose).
Sugar	Fructose. Garnish desserts with puréed or stewed fruit. Finely chop dried fruit and add to cereals, porridge, yoghurt, cakes, pie bases and sweet and sour dishes. Use mashed banana on cereals. Use a little raw honey instead of sugar in hot drinks.
Colas	Herbal drink (for example, Aqualibra, Amé) or juice mixed 50–50 with sparkling water.
Chocolate	Low-sugar muesli bar, carob bar, fruit bar, dried fruit.

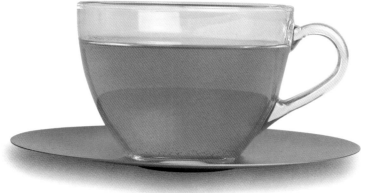

Neuro-lymphatic pressure points

Traditional Chinese medicine states that invisible channels, called meridians, run through the body. Energy (known as qi or chi) flows through these. Proper breathing is crucial to boosting qi levels. To enhance your breathing skills see page 132. If the flow of energy is blocked along the meridians, it can lead to health problems. Blockages can be released by stimulating certain points on the meridians through acupuncture. Neuro-lymphatic points, some of which are illustrated here, may also be used for acupressure. Using these points in conjunction with muscle testing (see page 122) is fascinating and during therapy the therapist will often use the points to "strengthen" muscles which respond weakly to testing. In this way, it can be ascertained if the energy flows have been unblocked to allow qi to circulate along the meridians.

There is no need to visit a therapist or use needles. You apply a rubbing pressure to the point to help reorganize energy flows. At first, it is usual for the points to be quite uncomfortable when they are rubbed – some people say that the more the points hurt, the more the therapy is needed. Do not rub skin that is bruised or broken. If you have any of the problems illustrated on the following pages, work on the relevant point to relieve the disorder.

Chinese medicine views health as pertaining to the body, the mind and the spirit. Responses to treatment are studied on many levels, not just the physical and the philosophy is the same for muscle testing, which incorporates many principles of Chinese medicine. By addressing these points you can have a direct impact on particular problems but there is also a greater impact on general health by the unblocking of qi energy. In ancient times, Chinese physicians were paid as long as the patient was healthy. Once the person fell ill all further medicines and treatments were free of charge. Perhaps we can learn from this principle!

HEADACHES

GALL BLADDER MERIDIAN

Point 31 (GB31)

To find GB31, stand with your arms at your side. Where your middle finger touches your leg on your trouser seam is the point. Rub GB31 on both legs to melt your headaches away.

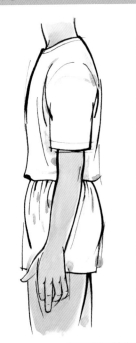

TOXICITY AND BOWEL HEALTH

LARGE INTESTINE MERIDIAN

Point 4 (LI4)

To find LI4, pinch the area between your thumb and index finger where the skin is webbed, by using the thumb and index finger of the opposite hand. Go towards the joint and rub. Do the same to the other hand. This point is called "The Great Eliminator" in Chinese medicine. Do not use this technique if you are pregnant.

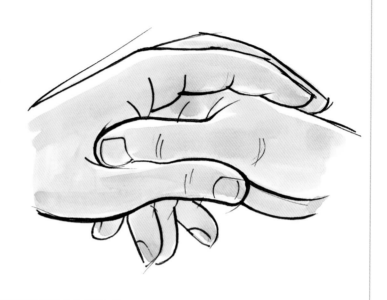

CLUMSINESS AND CONFUSION

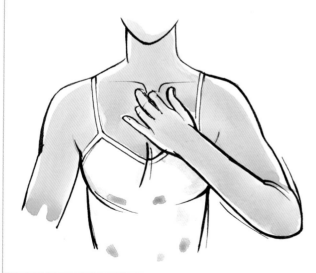

KIDNEY MERIDIAN

Point 27 (K27)

This point is a master point through which all the meridians flow. For this reason it is very effective for "neurological disorganization". To find K27, locate the peaks of your clavicle (collarbone) at the base of your throat with the index finger and thumb of one hand. Let your fingertips drop into the hollows just below the two peaks. You can also rub your navel with your opposite hand for maximum effect.

Muscle testing

Muscle testing, or kinesiology, is a fascinating treatment option for a number of disorders, including muscular and emotional problems. But one of its most interesting uses is for testing for food intolerances. Kinesiology uses a mixture of chiropractic muscle response tests and Chinese medicine diagnosis of energy flow in the meridians. To test for food reactions, what is generally looked for is a weak muscle response to foods that offend and a strong muscle response to foods that are helpful. A qualified therapist will look for more subtle reactions, which describe complex situations such as the interaction between a number of foods. However, here is a simple experiment you can use at home to test how foods, and even thoughts, might affect you.

MUSCLE TESTING

1 You will need another person to help you. Do not attempt this if you have back, neck or shoulder problems. Put both arms up at your sides, at shoulder height, so that you form a T-shape.

2 Your friend (who is standing facing you) must now place a hand above each of your wrists, slightly over the long bones of the arm and not the hand, and say "Hold" whilst exerting slight downward pressure in order to try and collapse your arms. You should be able to hold the stance and meet the pressure. This is not a test of strength and you will either be able to hold the position or you will not. Practise a couple of times to get the feel of the test.

3 Next, after resting your arms for a moment, ask your friend to put a little sugar on your tongue and then immediately perform the test again. The majority of people will find that their arms are not able to resist the pressure, indicating that the sugar is somehow interfering with their correct body functioning.

4 Retest by repeating step three without the sugar (wash your mouth out with water).

5 You can try this experiment again with thoughts. First, think of something pleasant and then do the test. Try it again with an unhappy thought, then switch back to a nice thought. Instead of sugar, foods such as coffee, bread, cheese or chocolate can be substituted for testing.

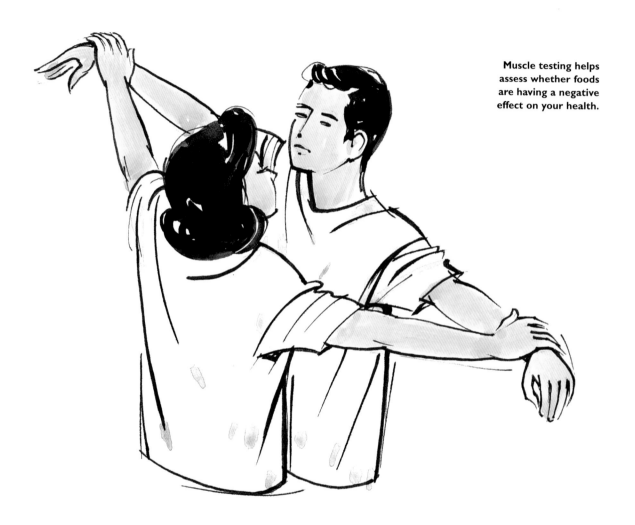

Muscle testing helps assess whether foods are having a negative effect on your health.

Life is like a wild tiger. You can either lie down and let it lay its paw on your head, or sit on its back and ride.

TRANSLATED FROM "RIDE THE WILD TIGER"

Feeling fit

Humans are designed to move, but many of us lead very sedentary lives. It is not necessary to spend hours in the gym to get fit, but you do need to use your body in the way that nature intended. We were not designed to travel to work in a car, sit in an office for eight hours, and collapse in a heap in front of the television at the end of the day. In the 20 years from 1975 to 1995, the annual distance that the average person walked fell from 410 kilometres (255 miles) to 320 kilometres (200 miles) a year – a drop of 20 per cent.

We are suffering from a lethargy epidemic. All the devices that make our lives easier, such as washing machines, vacuum cleaners and TV remote controls, also rob us of valuable body-moving opportunities. But making small changes to your routine can pay immense dividends. Try walking briskly to work, or getting off the bus or train early and walking at least a few blocks. Take the stairs instead of the lift. Carry the groceries back from the shops instead of using the car. All these efforts will help to burn up hundreds of extra calories daily. Just climbing five flights of stairs every day will significantly lower your risk of heart disease. If you walked an extra kilometre a day, without changing your food intake, you would lose 2.7kg (6lb) in a year.

Physical activity can clear your mind and assist in keeping stress under control by helping to remove adrenaline from the blood. Exercise also causes the release of endorphins (the body's natural feel-good hormones). It helps to increase the motility of the colon and to resolve constipation, which in turn encourages the body to detoxify. Exercise helps to normalize women's hormone levels, and there is evidence to suggest that women who exercise regularly have considerably fewer problems with PMS, the menopause and breast cancer when compared to women who do not exercise. Exercise increases oxygen consumption, and this is believed to be the reason why taking up sport can significantly improve the health of people who suffer from panic attacks or agoraphobia.

TO BURN 100 CALORIES YOU NEED TO:

Walk at 4 kph (2.5 mph) for 20 minutes.

Weed the garden for 22 minutes.

Wash the dishes or clean the house for

28 minutes.

Wash the car or sweep floors for 30 minutes.

Vacuum for 38 minutes.

Do the ironing for 50 minutes.

Sit and read or watch TV for 105 minutes.

Sleep for 120 minutes.

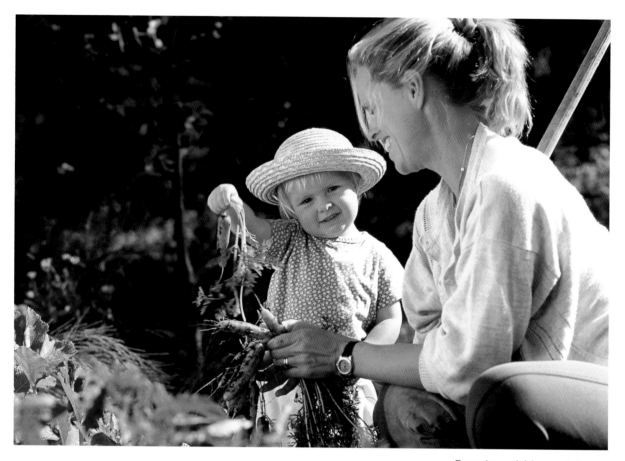

Everyday activities can help you become fitter without realizing it. Weeding the garden for 22 minutes, for example, burns up 100 calories.

If you have difficulty sleeping, exercising is one of the best ways of ensuring a good night's sleep. Do not exercise just before going to bed, because it is too much of a stimulant, but you can do relaxation exercises in the evening to help you become drowsy.

The benefits of exercise to the cardiovascular system are huge. A cardiovascular work-out will improve the strength of your heart muscle. Relaxation exercises fight stress, which is one of the biggest risk factors for cardiovascular problems.

To get the maximum benefit for your heart and to burn up the most body fat, you need to exercise at an intensity that raises your pulse rate and gets you warm, but does not make you so out of breath that you cannot hold a conversation. This represents about 75 per cent of your maximum working capacity, which is the best fat-burning range to operate in. Drink plenty of water to avoid dehydration. There is no great need to calculate your pulse rate, but if you do, you can monitor your increasing fitness by noting how much your pulse rate drops over time.

FITNESS FORMULA

You can check your fitness by working out your recovery rate after exercise.

1. Take your pulse for 15 seconds and multiply by four to get the number of beats in a minute. Do this immediately after stopping exercising, and then again a minute later.

2. Subtract the second figure from the first and divide by ten. Therefore, if your pulse was 140 when you stopped, and 100 a minute later, the calculation would be: $140 - 100 = 40$. $40 \div 10 = 4$.

3. Check your fitness level against the chart.

Less than 2	Poor
2–3	Fair
3–4	Good
4–6	Excellent
Greater than 6	Athlete level

Always warm up before exercise and cool down afterwards. Build up to your full intensity slowly to avoid pulling any muscles. If you have a pre-existing cardiovascular problem, osteoporosis or any other serious health concerns, it is best to check with your doctor before starting an exercise programme. Methods of warming up and cooling down include walking on the spot for three or four minutes, and doing stretches of all the major muscle groups, particularly the leg muscles.

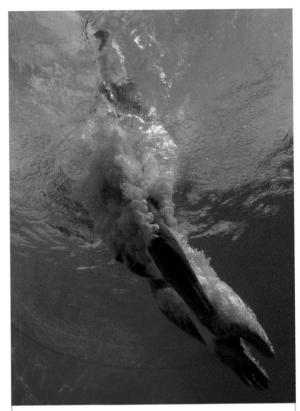

EXERCISE CHOICES

Cycling, swimming, water aerobics, fast walking, dance These rhythmic activities also give you a cardiovascular work-out. They are appropriate for people who want to exercise on their own at a time that is convenient, with the minimum of equipment and instruction. You also have an excuse to take advantage of fine weather with cycling and walking, and dancing means that you can listen to great music at the same time! Swimming supports 90 per cent of your body weight, virtually eliminating the potential for impact injury. Water aerobics uses the fact that water is 800 times more dense than air, creating a resistance similar to working with weights.

EXERCISE CHOICES

Yoga, Tai Chi, Pilates, Psychocalisthenics™, Callanetics These options are slow and have a meditative quality. Many of these systems focus on energy centres and have a strong therapeutic element to them. Find out about classes near you, or if necessary buy a video.

Home gym This suits people who want to work out at home. There is no need for classes (though it is important to learn to use equipment correctly). It is perfect for those who want to exercise at different times.

Tennis, rowing, football These sports will help you to learn about co-operation, and being in a team helps with motivation.

Aerobics, jogging, circuit training High-intensity activities to suit those who are fairly fit and energetic, though you can work at your own speed and build up your fitness level.

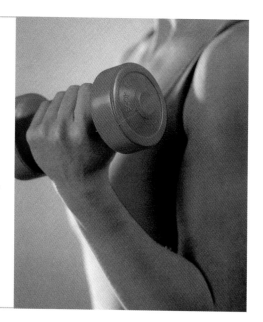

REBOUNDER EXERCISES

A rebounder is a mini-trampoline designed for home use. It can be stored under a bed. Buy a model with six legs for stability. Rebounding has several benefits. Because you are working against gravity, lymph is pushed around the lymph channels, giving an extra boost to the cleansing of your system. Rebounding is a low-impact exercise and is very gentle on the joints. Because bouncing is fun, it does not really feel like exercise and helps lift the spirits.

Basic bounce

Bouncing on the spot is a good introduction to rebounding. You get all the benefits of lymph being moved around your body, which helps detoxification.

Let's twist again

Increase the bouncing and use your arms. Twist at the waist, moving arms and hips in opposite directions.

Ski-slope slalom

Keep your ankles together as you take small sideways jumps, as if you were dodging round slalom poles when skiing down a mountain. Your arms swing back and forth in opposition.

Jogging on the spot

Jogging can be done at different speeds. Increase the intensity by pumping your arms, or by kicking your legs behind you. Another variation is to do knee lifts.

Jumping jacks

This is high-intensity rebounding, where you jump and kick your arms and legs out at the same time. You can do jumping jacks to the side, bringing your arms up to shoulder height, or forwards and backwards, moving your arms back and forth in opposition.

STRETCHES

Stretches can be used to relieve stress, or as a warm-up before more rigorous exercise. If you do not have the energy or time to do a full work-out or a complete relaxation or meditation routine, doing a few stretches for five or ten minutes will bring great rewards. If you stretch and stay supple, your musculature and mind will benefit. With advancing years, many people "seize up" and daily stretches are the best way to ensure that this never happens. Use it or lose it! You can do the stretches almost anywhere, but do aim to get five minutes' peace while you practise them.

The cat

● Kneel on all fours with your hands and knees shoulder-width apart. Breathe in and then as you exhale, lift and arch your back and tuck your head and your tail down. Hold for a moment, in a deep stretch, before returning to your original position. Breathe in, then on the out-breath, reverse the movement – create a hollow in your back and tilt your tail up, with your head back. Return to your original position.

Leg stretches

● Stand up holding the back of a chair or the edge of a table, bend one knee and place the other leg 60cm (2ft) behind you, with the sole of your foot on the floor. You will feel a stretch at the back of the knee of the extended leg. Hold for a count of 20. Repeat with the other leg.

● Now, steadying yourself with one hand, use the other hand to pull your leg up behind you. Feel a stretch in your front thigh muscle. If you can, extend the leg a little further behind you by pulling it outwards with your hand. Repeat the movement with the other leg.

● Sit on the floor with your legs in front of you and your feet together. Clasp your calves, ankles or feet with your hands and pull your body forwards so that your head goes towards your feet. Hold for a count of 20.

● Remain on the floor, extend one leg in front of you, and tuck the heel of the other leg into your groin, or as far as you can get it. Bend over, pointing your nose towards your knees. Hold for a count of 20. Repeat with the other leg. Do not worry if you do not get very far with these stretches to start with, you will find that after a few sessions you gradually become more supple.

Arm, shoulder and neck stretches

● Stand tall and with one hand, reach over your shoulder to the middle of your shoulder blades. Increase the stretch by gently applying pressure to your elbow with the other hand. Hold for a count of 20 and then repeat with the other arm.

● Now clasp your hands behind you, interlocking your fingers, then stretch your arms and feel the stretch in your upper back and shoulders. Hold for a count of 20.

● Finally, arch your neck forward, allowing your chin to drop on to your chest. Very slowly, circle your head to look over one shoulder, then roll it back to your starting position. Do not tense up. Repeat in the other direction. Perform the movement twice more in each direction.

I am a part of all that I have met.

ALFRED, LORD TENNYSON

TOP FIVE EXERCISE TIPS

1 Choose a means of exercising that you really enjoy. Exercise is not meant to be endured: it should be fun.

2 Remember that three spells of exercise for ten minutes each, daily, is just as beneficial as one session lasting 30 minutes.

3 Take an antioxidant supplement 30 minutes before starting vigorous exercise. This can help to reduce the effects of oxidation damage to tissues. Antioxidant supplements usually contain vitamins A, C and E, and the minerals selenium and zinc.

4 Keep hydrated. Always drink a large glass of water before you exercise, and one just after. If you are thirsty during exercise, top up with more water. The dehydration of a muscle by a mere three per cent leads to a 10 per cent reduction in muscle tensile strength.

5 Pump up the volume and dance! It makes you feel good, and is terrific all-round aerobic exercise.

Stress-busting weekends

What do you use your weekends for? Relaxing, recharging your batteries and enjoying yourself? Perhaps you catch up on unfinished work, clean the house, and do all the things you haven't had time for during the week? Or do you collapse in an immovable stupor? Here are some ideas for how to make the most of your weekends and do some real stress-busting.

ENERGY-BOOSTING TIPS

■ On Friday evening, go out and enjoy yourself instead of slumping in front of the television. Going out on a Friday night helps to make your weekends seem longer – more of a mini-break. It is the quickest way to switch your thoughts from the cares of the week to relaxation. If you have time to have a bath before you go out, add a handful of dried rosemary and a little sea salt to the bathwater. It will help you feel fresh and energized. Get to bed by midnight.

■ Don't oversleep in the morning. Keeping to a regular schedule helps to preserve energy levels.

■ Get your chores done early on Saturday. Decide what needs to be done, allot a specific time and when the time is up, stop! The rest of the weekend is yours.

■ Farm out the children for a few hours on one day. There are two days to the weekend – it is not necessary to feel guilty if you keep part of one of those days for yourself.

■ Wear bright colours. Colours can affect your mood: yellow and orange are energizing, while white, blue, purple and green are calming.

WEEKEND 1
ENERGY-BOOSTING PLAN

A change is as good as a rest. In order to greet Monday with a smile, concentrate on an energy-boosting weekend.

EAT FOR VITALITY

The main message for this weekend is to keep it simple. Eat light meals, at least half of which should be raw fruit, raw vegetables, nuts and seeds – all powerhouses of nutrients. Experiment with new dishes that include raw foods such as soups, purées, dips and patés. Juicing is an excellent way of obtaining revitalizing nutrients and beneficial food enzymes, and juice drinks make good mid-morning and afternoon snacks. If you don't have a juicer, whizz organic fruit juice and fresh soft fruit together in a blender.

Friday evening

● A salad, followed by fish or chicken and vegetables. Or a stir-fry with lots of vegetables.

● Herbal tea. No dessert, but you may have a square or two of 70% cocoa solid chocolate.

● Alcohol. By all means have a drink if it helps you to relax, but do not overdo it and drink equal measures of water. White drinks (white wine, vodka and gin) contain fewer

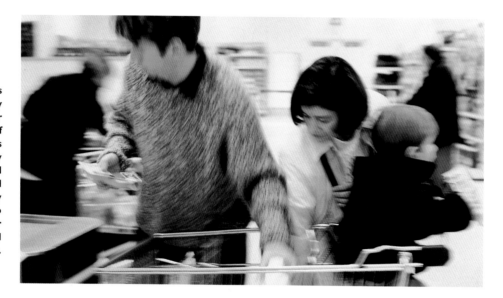

Assign chores to Saturday morning. After that, the rest of the weekend is your own. Buy lots of fruit and vegetables, and other healthy ingredients, to cleanse your system and and increase vitality.

compounds that promote headaches and hangovers than darker drinks (red wine, whisky and brandy).

Saturday and Sunday
Breakfast
Your body needs refuelling: complex carbohydrates are best for this, so choose from a bowl of porridge, wholemeal toast, oatcakes or wholegrain muesli (wheat-free if avoiding wheat).

Snack – mid-morning and mid-afternoon
● A freshly prepared fruit or vegetable juice.

Lunch
A salad or soup with a difference, for instance:
● Tuna and chickpea salad with chopped cherry tomatoes, basil and chives.
● Sprouted beans, lentils, sweetcorn, tomatoes, red onion and tahini, garlic and lemon juice dressing.
● Gazpacho soup.
● Cooked lentils with fresh plum tomatoes and mint.
● Split pea and courgette soup with sesame seeds.

● Spicy bean soup.
● If you are very hungry, add toasted pumpernickel bread or pitta bread stuffed with houmous and salad.

Evening meal
On Saturday, the ingredients double up as skincare.
● Oily fish, such as salmon, with a salad of lettuce, avocado and cucumber, dressed with walnut oil and lemon juice. Make a dessert with oatmeal, chopped strawberries and yoghurt.
● After a warm bath, scrub your face with some oatmeal in yoghurt to slough off dead skin. Rub walnut oil on your body, concentrating on the dry parts. Apply a mashed avocado and strawberry face-mask, pop a couple of cucumber slices on your eyes, lie down and relax. Remember to put a towel over the bed to prevent the oil staining the covers.
● On Sunday, follow the instructions for Friday evening.

Before bed
● An oatmeal drink or cereal drink such as barley cup made with warm soya milk sweetened with honey.

DE-STRESSING TIPS

■ Prepare ahead. In fact, start preparing for the weekend three days in advance.

■ Plan. List everything you need to do for a successful weekend. Make shopping lists, activity plans, seating arrangements. Find tools for the job, favourite music to relax to, clothes that make you feel good.

■ Delegate. If the list looks unwieldy, cut it back to what is practicable. Ask others to lend a hand. Cut out unnecessary tasks – if you are entertaining, don't overstretch yourself by straining to whisk up a perfect soufflé if a paté you have already bought will do just as well for a starter.

■ Stress protection nutrients. If you are not already doing so, take anti-stress nutrients to help make sure your reserves are not depleted in the days to come: 50mg B-complex, 2g vitamin C in two divided doses,

■ 15mg zinc and 500mg magnesium.

■ Relax on Friday evening. Have a long soak in the bath, crank up the music, dim the lights and sip a relaxing herbal infusion. Or go for an invigorating walk, vowing to take in details you don't usually notice, such as the shapes of leaves, or the sounds of birds.

■ Over the weekend, take your mind on regular, 15-minute brain holidays, at least once every two hours. Set an alarm if you need reminding, find a quiet corner, and lie or sit comfortably. Imagine all the lovely things you are going to do for yourself next week, or remember an enjoyable experience, or just drift off to a place that makes you happy.

■ Incorporate relaxation and breathing exercises into your day. Allowing just five minutes for this can make all the difference to managing well.

WEEKEND 2
DE-STRESSING PLAN:
FOR COPING WITH AN UNAVOIDABLY HECTIC WEEKEND

When the approaching weekend is looming with challenges, such as a visit from the in-laws, eight people for lunch, a project to finish, the spare room to decorate, or your child's birthday party to cater for, here is a plan to help you come out of the other end – sane!

EAT TO PREVENT STRESS

● Start well on the Saturday. Give your body a treat with a health-giving breakfast to set yourself up for the rest of the day. Make an exotic fruit salad (choose from pineapple, papaya, avocado, pomegranate, pear, kiwi fruit, blueberries, dried apple slices or anything else that takes your fancy). Top with live yoghurt or fresh orange juice and add some chopped fresh nuts.

● Enjoy eating with your friends and family, but don't eat or drink too much. Ensure that socialising does not mean an increase in your consumption of caffeine and sugar.

RELAXATION AND BREATHING

It is not always easy to relax when you are feeling tense. One way to help the process is to focus completely on another activity. We take breathing for granted (and it is not normally under our conscious control), however if we focus on it, it is hard to worry about anything else. This is how to relax and breathe well.

● Find a quiet and comfortable place to sit (or to lie).
● With your feet slightly apart, place one hand on your navel, and the other on your chest.
● Inhale through your nose and exhale through your mouth.

● Concentrate on your breathing, and notice which hand is rising and falling with your in- and out-breaths.

● Gently breathe out most of the air in your lungs.

● Inhale slowly, while counting to four.

● As you inhale, allow your abdomen to rise slightly, but do not hunch or tense your shoulders at the same time.

● As you breathe in, imagine the warmed air flowing into your lungs and from there into all parts of your body.

● Pause for a second, and then slowly exhale to a count of four. As you exhale, your abdomen should drop.

● Imagine all the stresses, anxieties and tensions leaving your body as you exhale.

I wish that I was where I am.

GERTRUDE STEIN

JUICING IDEAS

Make yourself a delicious drink packed with vitamins and minerals.
Pop the ingredients into a blender and whizz together for a few minutes.

APPLE-BASED DRINKS

■ 1 apple, 3 sticks celery, 25g (1oz) parsley.

■ 1 apple, 15 pitted cherries.

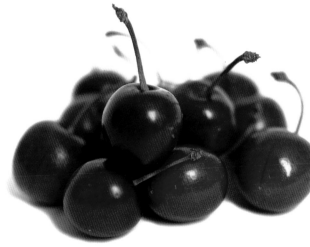

CITRUS-BASED DRINKS

■ 1 grapefruit, ¼ melon, ground cinnamon.

■ 1 orange, 1 lime, 2 carrots, 2.5cm (1in) cube of ginger root.

TOMATO-BASED DRINKS

■ 3 tomatoes, 1 clove garlic, 1 stick celery.

■ 2 tomatoes, handful of watercress, ¼ cucumber.

WINTER VEGETABLE DRINKS

■ 3 carrots, 6 spinach leaves, 100g (4oz) red cabbage.

■ ½ cauliflower, ½ leek, 2 sticks celery, 1 carrot.

■ 1 green pepper, ½ head fennel, ¼ beetroot, 1 carrot

WEEKEND 3
DETOX PLAN

Use this weekend to cleanse your system, and start the following week feeling fresh and energized.

Our bodies are super-efficient at dealing with toxins. The liver processes them, and lymph and blood carry them away to be disposed of through the skin, lungs, kidneys and colon. This system works well as long as the body is not overloaded by toxins; however, when it is continually under assault by chemicals, pesticides and processed foods, it is easy for an excess of toxins to build up. Signs of toxicity include feeling tired all the time, cellulite, bad breath, coated tongue, headaches, migraines, spots, aching joints, cloudy urine and irregular bowel movements.

A weekend detoxification plan, undertaken once a month, can go a long way to revitalizing you. Of course, detoxification – detoxing – should be regarded as a long-term approach to promoting health, but devoting a weekend to "spring cleaning" is a good place to start. Measures such as drinking lots of pure water, and making fresh, vitamin-packed juices can eventually be incorporated into your daily routine. External treatments, such as dry skin brushing, can also be added to your future body maintenance plan.

LIFESTYLE DETOX TIPS

■ Friday lunchtime. Make a shopping list of items you need for the weekend. Check the newspaper entertainment listings for anything you may want to do over the weekend, because from now on newspapers are banned until Monday morning.

■ Let daylight wake you up naturally instead of using an alarm clock.

■ Avoid watching television, opening the post, using the internet or reading the newspapers for the whole weekend. Instead take the opportunity to do something you do not usually do, such as a brisk walk, swimming, visiting a new exhibition, or reading a good, non-stressful book.

■ Do 15–30 minutes of relaxation exercises or meditation.

■ Do a dry skin brush (see page 136) before a warm bath, using your choice of aromatherapy oils.

■ Get to bed by 10pm on Friday, Saturday and Sunday – it's luxury!

■ Dispose of some clutter over the weekend. Clear out your handbag, a shelf or a box filled with accumulated bits and pieces.

■ Allocate time to "Detox Your Mind" (see *Visualization*, page 141).

■ Do not eat your evening meals after 7.30 pm Plan to eat between 6 pm and 7 pm

EAT TO DETOX

All food you eat this weekend will be free of the substances that are most likely to clutter up your system. By avoiding them, your body has a chance to throw off accumulated toxins. Do not have processed foods, alcohol, coffee, tea, other sources of caffeine, wheat, dairy products, and animal protein (if you find this last step too difficult, you may eat a little fish or skinless organic chicken).

If you find that you experience headaches, a furred tongue, an increased need to urinate, or other unexpected symptoms, it is likely to signify that your body is in urgent need of this detoxification programme. Drink plenty of water throughout the weekend – a minimum of two litres of water each day. Water is ideally either filtered, good-quality mineral water, or distilled water. In addition to the two litres of water, if you want a hot drink, chamomile, valerian and vervain teas are ideal.

Friday evening

Start your detox weekend on Friday evening. The menu is the same as the choices listed for Saturday and Sunday.

Saturday and Sunday

Just after rising, drink some hot water with freshly squeezed lemon juice.

Breakfast

A juice of your choice (see page 133 for ideas) and either:
● Home-made muesli made from rice flakes, roasted buckwheat groats, millet flakes, sunflower seeds, soaked prunes and their juice and grated apple.
● Millet porridge made from millet flakes. Top with dried fruit, seeds and apple juice.
● Rice puffs (sugar-free and low-salt) with rice milk and banana slices.

Snacks

● Fresh fruit and unsulphured dried fruit. Pumpkin seeds are also helpful for cleansing the digestive tract.

Lunch

● Vegetable stir-fry, with brown rice sprinkled with sesame seeds.
● A large baked potato stuffed with houmous and a freshly made coleslaw salad (grated white cabbage, carrot and onion, dressed with olive oil and cider vinegar).
● Chickpea and tomato curry, served with wholegrain basmati rice. To make the curry, fry some onion and garlic in a tiny bit of olive oil (or steam-fry in water). Add curry paste along with a teaspoonful of cumin, which is rich in the powerful plant compound curcumin. Put in a can of drained and rinsed chickpeas and a can of tomatoes. Stir and simmer for 15 minutes so that the flavours meld together.

Pre-dinner drink

● Before your evening meal, drink the juice of half a lemon diluted in a cup of hot water.

Evening meal

● In summer, have a large salad made from a selection of the following foods, choosing at least one herb or vegetable from each of the eight groups. Dress your salad with lemon juice, olive oil and garlic.

Leaves: dandelion, watercress, lettuce, cabbage, spinach, cress.
Herbs: coriander, basil, parsley, thyme, mint.
Onions: spring onions, chives, red onion, white onion.

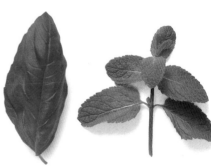

Winter selection: raw cauliflower, carrots, broccoli, beetroot.

Summer selection: tomato, peppers (any colour) radishes, cucumber, celery.

Beans and peas: mangetout, chickpeas, any beans, any sprouted beans.

Seeds and nuts: pumpkin seeds, sesame seeds, sunflower seeds, hemp seeds, walnuts, almonds, brazil nuts.

Other: olives, bamboo shoots, water chestnuts.

● In winter you may want a more warming meal, such as soup. Choose from the following, unless you have ideas of your own:

■ Parsnip, pumpkin, coriander and ginger.

■ Vegetable soup with a "kick" (mixed vegetables and cayenne pepper).

■ Thai garlic and shiitaki (French onion soup base with shiitaki mushrooms, lemon grass and garlic). Sprinkle with plenty of chopped parsley.

Finish your meal with a fruit salad, including chopped fresh nuts and dried fruit, and moisten it with the juice of a freshly squeezed orange. Some good combinations are:

■ Mandarin and peach with fresh grated ginger and toasted flaked almonds.

■ Papaya and kiwi fruit with chopped hazelnuts.

■ Pineapple and mango with roughly chopped brazil nuts.

■ Honeydew melon and raspberries.

■ Prune and apricot compôte with walnuts.

■ Strawberries, stewed rhubarb, roasted sunflower seeds.

■ Blackcurrant, apple and chopped almonds.

■ Watermelon (and eat the crunchy seeds for the detoxifying potassium they contain).

Bedtime drink

■ Make a liver-cleansing herbal tea with dandelion, ginger, lemon and half a teaspoonful of honey, or drink a mixture of

DRY SKIN BRUSHING

One of the best ways of getting rid of toxins is to brush your skin. Buy a natural bristle body brush, and keep it solely for this purpose.

Before your bath or shower, on dry skin, spend five minutes brushing with long, sweeping motions from your toes upwards. Brush the soles of your feet, moving on to your whole body. Brush from your fingertips and the palms of your hands, towards your heart. Avoid brushing any broken skin, or your nipples. When you step into the bath or shower, you will be tingling all over.

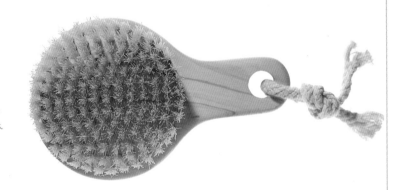

Skin brushing loosens dead skin cells, but more importantly it improves blood and lymph flow just below the surface of the skin. This in turn stimulates all your detoxification systems to eliminate toxins more efficiently.

CLEAR OUT YOUR CLUTTER

When you go on holiday, you pack a few items that mix and match, giving you many potential outfits. But faced with a wardrobe crammed with the last 15 years' purchases, you cannot decide what to wear. The choice was easier, and more successful, when you had less to choose from.

In the same way, clutter makes other aspects of life more difficult. A cluttered desk will hide valuable information and mask priorities. A cluttered room will not be a relaxing place to be. A cluttered life will be chaotic and stressful.

Set aside one hour, a couple of times a week, to have a clear-out. Follow these rules for assessing your possessions:

Use it, or:
Mend it immediately and use it, or:
File it straight away, properly labelled, if there is a reason for keeping it, or:
Get rid of it.

Go through your post and deal with it every day. Pay bills when they come in – if they pile up they will be another source of stress to wear you down. Go through your wardrobe once every six months and get rid of items you have not worn. Keep up to date with jobs such as sewing on buttons and getting clothes dry-cleaned. Clearing clutter is an essential part of detoxing your mind and body.

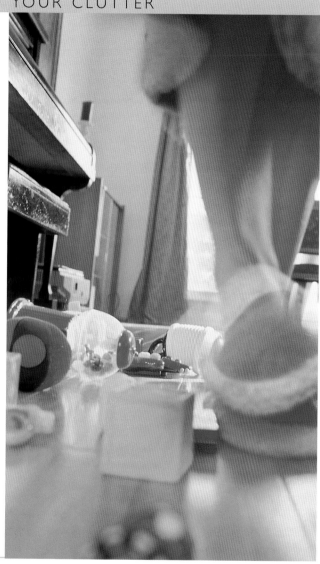

A man there was, though some did count him mad,

The more he cast away, the more he had.

JOHN BUNYAN

Stress-busting week plan

To deal with stress effectively, we need to eat a nutrient-dense diet with sufficient protein to repair tissues and to balance brain chemicals, and to avoid stimulants. It is important to eat foods that do not cause any adverse reactions. As you address your diet, you will become more aware of foods that do not agree with you.

For people who are regularly under stress, meals that balance proteins with carbohydrates are ideal. The proteins do not have to come from animal sources such as meat or fish – plant sources include nuts, soya, beans, lentils and seeds. Meals that combine complex carbohydrates with tryptophan-rich foods (see page 22) help stabilize levels of the brain chemical serotonin. If serotonin levels are out of balance, addictions to sugar, alcohol, coffee, refined carbohydrates or other stimulants can worsen.

TIPS FOR YOUR STRESS-BUSTING WEEK

Each day invest 1$\frac{1}{2}$ hours in yourself:

■ Do something pleasurable such as buying yourself flowers, reading a glossy magazine, or having a massage, sauna or a manicure.

■ Take vitamins, skin brush before your bath and moisturize afterwards.

■ Do at least 30 minutes of exercise. It doesn't have to be energetic – you could go for a walk in the park.

■ Listen to a relaxation tape for 20 minutes, meditate or do some yoga.

■ Get into the habit of using one of the following stress-busting techniques: "Visualization" (see page 141), "Emotional Release Technique" (see page 141), or "Walk Tall" (see page 143).

■ At the end of the day, reflect on all the positive things that you have achieved, and what you have learned. Remember, even if you have had a bad day, you will have learned something from it.

During the week:

■ Plan an enjoyable event for some time in the future and reserve this time in your diary now. It could be a visit, a holiday, a party, a weekend away, a visit to a health farm, or even a parachuting course.

EAT TO BALANCE BRAIN CHEMICALS

Breakfast choices

Begin your breakfast with freshly squeezed fruit or vegetable juice, or a portion of fruit, then enjoy one of the following:

- Oatcakes with nut butter (such as almond, cashew, peanut) or mackerel paté.
- Baked beans on rye toast.
- Porridge and seeds with milk or soya milk.
- Muesli and red berries with skimmed milk or soya milk.
- Boiled egg with Ryvita crackers.
- Soya yoghurt and chopped banana, sprinkled with mixed spice.
- Grilled unsmoked bacon (all visible fat trimmed) and mushrooms.
- Baked kipper and grilled tomatoes.

Light meal choices

- Cottage cheese and chopped spring onion sandwich, or cottage cheese and peach slices on rye crackers.
- Jacket potato with baked beans and coleslaw.
- Thick lentil soup.
- Mixed sprouted bean salad.
- Smoked mackerel with tomato and avocado salad.
- Turkey and salad sandwich, made with rye bread.
- Broccoli and cauliflower cheese.
- Scrambled egg with smoked salmon pieces and wholemeal toast.
- Sardines on rye toast, served with a green salad.

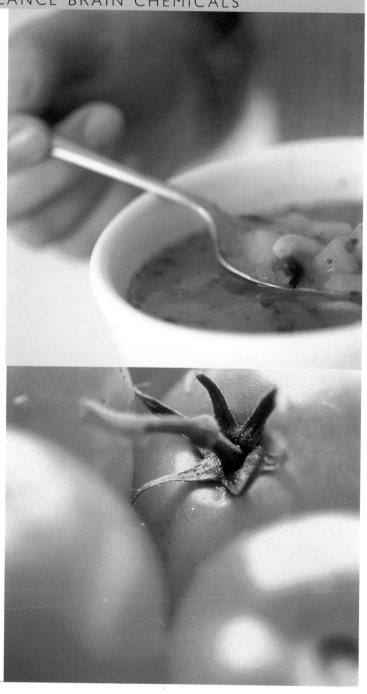

EAT TO BALANCE BRAIN CHEMICALS

Main meal choices

- Game casserole served with red cabbage, baked celeriac and mashed potato.
- Chickpea, kidney bean and flageolet bean stew made with tomatoes, red and yellow peppers, aubergines, mushrooms, onions and garlic, with wholewheat or corn pasta.
- Poached salmon with new potatoes and stir-fried julienned (cut into thin strips) vegetables with ginger.
- Bean, potato and spinach curry served with brown rice and raita (yoghurt with grated onion and cucumber).
- Turkey breast with green beans, sliced carrots and chestnut and sage stuffing balls.
- Canneloni bean casserole, spinach, smoked tofu and brown rice.
- Tofu and Mediterranean roasted vegetables on a bed of polenta.
- Seafood provençal (prawns, mussels, octopus rings, firm white fish in tomato and herbs) with buckwheat pasta.

Snack choices

Eat snacks between meals to keep your blood sugar levels even. Good options are:

- Carrot sticks dipped in houmous.
- Fresh fruit with plain yoghurt or chopped nuts or seeds.
- Nuts and seeds.
- A few tortilla crisps dipped in dhal (dip made from lentils and garlic).
- Small square of cheese and half an apple.
- Small mixed salad with pine nuts.
- Natural yoghurt (soya or dairy) with fruit.
- Celery sticks stuffed with taramasalata.
- Left-overs from lunch or evening meal.
- Boiled egg and an oatcake.
- Sprouted beans and pulses.

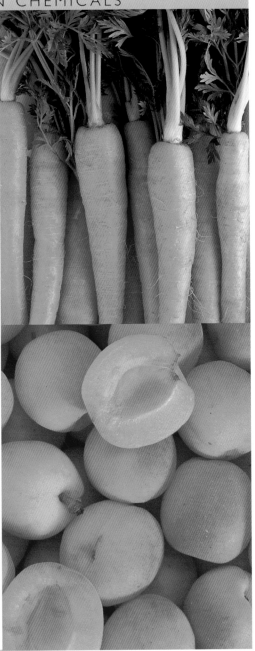

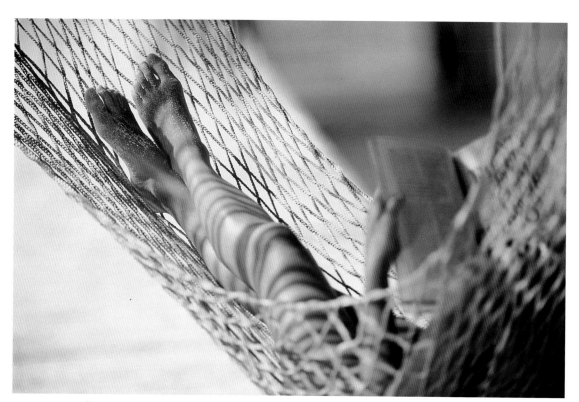

Keep a vision of a perfect environment in your memory and revisit it when you are feeling stressed.

EMOTIONAL RELEASE TECHNIQUE

This very simple technique has great results.

● Place the index and middle finger of each hand on your forehead about 2.5cm (1in) above the eyebrows.

● Gently hold these energy points and tug the skin upwards very slightly.

● Close your eyes and think about something that is troubling you.

● Continue for several minutes, and you will usually find that it becomes more difficult to hold the thought and that stress ebbs away.

This method can even be effective for dealing with phobias. The effects are slightly more powerful if someone else touches the energy points for you. An advanced version of the technique is to touch the points with the thumb, index and middle finger of one hand while gently cupping the back of the head, where it meets the neck, with the other hand.

VISUALIZATION

We cannot see into the future, even if we wish that we could! We worry about what may or may not happen, but it does not serve any useful purpose. Instead, it is much better to think about your needs and plans. Most people don't get what they want because they do not have a clear idea of what it is. If you can smell, feel, hear and taste what you want – the chances of it becoming a reality are greater. This is visualization – a remarkable technique for changing your body and your responses to things.

● To do it, relax in a comfortable position, and make sure you are warm.
● Now turn your mind to what it is you want to change. For example, to banish feelings of stress you could imagine yourself lying on a beach – feel yourself bathed in warmth, with a gentle breeze playing on your skin, see the bright blue sky, smell the salty sea, hear waves washing back and forth.

● Take yourself back to this place every time you need to escape everyday worries.

Dramatic uses of visualization include imagining the taste of something you want to give up, say coffee, as unpalatable – perhaps tasting of something really disgusting. Work out your own ideas, but make sure that the associations are really strong. It is best to focus on one visualization message for several sessions, until it has made an impact, before you move on to the next one.

HOW FAR CAN YOU GO?

Experiment with this exercise, provided you do not have a bad back or other infirmity.

■ With your feet shoulder-width apart, aim to touch your toes without bending your knees.

■ Make a note of how far you managed to get.

■ Now stand up straight again and close your eyes. Without doing the actions, imagine you are touching your toes, and visualize yourself reaching further than you did before.

■ If you succeeded in touching your toes with your fingertips, imagine you are doing much better and putting the palms of your hands on the floor. Repeat the imagined exercise.

■ Now open your eyes and repeat the exercise for real. See what happens. Do not read on until you have done this exercise.

NOW READ THIS

Most people will find that they went much further the second time around. Why? You imagined yourself doing better, and so you did. It is as simple as that. When we imagine ourselves overcoming obstacles and achieving our aims, we find it much easier to do in reality. Visualize your successes and they will follow.

WALK TALL

It is impossible to feel down if you adopt the right posture. This is one of the exercises taught at drama classes.

First, sit or walk as if you are depressed. You probably hunch your shoulders and back, hang your head forward, shuffle your feet, breathe shallowly, and feel listless.

Now switch to a vibrant and positive stance. Throw your shoulders back, lift your head to look at a level slightly higher than straight ahead, walk or stand as though you feel happy and full of energy, and breathe deeply. How do you feel? Probably a lot better – or even great!

It is worth getting into the habit of checking your posture several times a day to remind yourself of how your stance is affecting your mood. After a few weeks, you will find that with improved posture, you are more confident and positive.

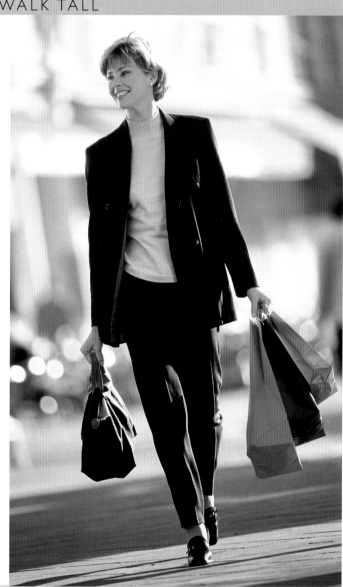

If you are too busy to laugh, you are too busy.

ANON

Stress-busting month plan

This plan is for those who are determined to make long-term changes to their eating habits and stress levels. It takes about a month to form new habits, such as changing a craving for sweet foods to a preference for those that are less sweet, losing the taste for salty foods, kicking the caffeine habit, passing the wine bottle without wavering, learning to be nice to yourself, and making significant improvements in your fitness levels. All these and more can be yours with this one-month plan – one month to change your life!

SOME ADVICE BEFORE YOU BEGIN

The Diet Tips are designed to be used for one month only. Do not be tempted to impose further diet restrictions on top of those suggested, and only do the fruit and vegetable cleanse on the stated days. Omit the cleansing days if you are pregnant or under a doctor's supervision for any reason. Do not drive or overtax yourself on designated cleansing days (switch them to another day if your plans cannot accommodate this). Enjoy experimenting with new foods throughout the plan. In addition to the Daily Self-Investment Tip, allocate at least 30 minutes a day as your own personal time and use it for a relaxation exercise (choose from visualization, meditation, or a breathing relaxation exercise), and daily stretches (see page 128).

DAY	DIET TIP (Add the day's tip to all the previous days' tips)	DAILY SELF-INVESTMENT TIP
1	From now until the end of the plan, drink two litres of water a day.	Read the tips for the next seven days and decide what plans you need to make and what you need to buy. Stock up on nutrient-rich foods (see page 74).
2	From now until the end of the plan, replace white flour products with wholegrain versions such as wholemeal bread, brown rice and wholewheat pasta.	Clear out some clutter: start with your handbag or the car.
3	Eat at least four pieces of fruit a day for the rest of the month. Add it to breakfast cereals, eat as a snack, and make into desserts.	Scalp massage (see page 148).

DAY	DIET TIP (Add the day's tip to all the previous days' tips)	DAILY SELF-INVESTMENT TIP
4	From now until the end of the month, avoid all sugar. Replace confectionery, cakes and biscuits with healthy options and snacks.	Rent a video for the evening – choose a comedy.
5	If you drink alcohol, resolve to only drink two measures, twice a week, from now on. If you can, avoid alcohol altogether for the rest of the month.	Check out what exercise classes are available locally, and the opening times of the swimming pool. Allocate time in your diary, twice a week, to do some energetic exercise.
6	Variety is the spice of life. When reorganizing your diet, don't be too restrictive. Make a list of all the foods you would like to try out during the next month.	If you have not yet bought some essential oils, do so today.
7	Go out for a meal and select something healthy, whether it is meat, fish, or pulses with vegetables. Make sure that at least one meal every day is really colourful (see "Stress-busting superfoods" on page 74).	Work out what arrangements you will need to make for the next week of the stress-busting plan, including items to buy.
8	From now until the end of the month, stop drinking tea and replace it with water, herbal tea or rooibos.	During the next few days you may feel tired and get headaches, because your body is detoxing. Take it easy and drink plenty of water.
9	From now until the end of the month, stop drinking coffee and replace it with water, caro, barley cup or dandelion coffee.	Go for a walk. Spend time reading an inspiring book, perhaps the biography of someone you admire.
10	From now on take a high dose multivitamin containing at least 50mg B-vitamins and 2000mg vitamin C divided into two doses.	Buy some flowers.
11	Eat a grain you have not tried before, such as buckwheat (pasta, noodles, flour for sauces, pancakes, roasted buckwheat).	Book a holiday, or weekend break, or organize a visit to a friend, for sometime in the near future.
12	From now until the end of the month (except when the day's diet tip specifies otherwise) replace wheat bread with oatcakes, 100 per cent rye bread, Ryvita, or homemade buckwheat pancakes.	Check your posture (see "Walk tall" on page 143).

DAY	DIET TIP (Add the day's tip to all the previous days' tips)	DAILY SELF-INVESTMENT TIP
13	Cook a meal (make up a recipe) using vegetables, beans, herbs and spices and wholewheat pasta, such as a stir-fry or spicy beans.	Indulge in a water therapy – your choice from page 100.
14	From now until the end of the month, start the day with freshly squeezed lemon juice and hot water.	Decide what arrangements you need to make and which items you need to buy for the next week of the plan.
15	CLEANSING DAY. Only eat vegetables today: salads, stir-fries, crudités and juices. Your digestion should be much improved by now, but if you have residual problems, follow the advice in "Stress and your digestive system" (page 44), particularly concerning juices, and use psyllium husks (buy from healthfood shops).	Skin brush and have a long bath with essential oils. Avoid newspapers, the internet and the TV today and tomorrow.
16	Avoid all wheat. Replace with rye, oats, barley, corn, potatoes, quinoa, buckwheat or millet.	Give yourself a face pack – you could combine it with your meal (see page 131)!
17	Make a recipe using tofu.	Make your evening meal special, by using candles, a tablecloth, best crockery and so on.
18	Until the end of the month, avoid all cheese and milk. Replace, if you need a replacement, with soya, rice milk or oat milk.	Clear out some clutter.
19	Eat another new grain, such as quinoa, polenta (corn) or barley pasta.	Have a scalp massage.
20	Make up a recipe (no recipe book) using raw foods only. Do not include lettuce.	Get a friend to do a reflexology relaxation session for you, then swap around (see page 51).
21	Include a new vegetable in your evening meal.	Plan ahead for the next week of the stress-busting plan.
22	Soak a handful of pulses in water overnight. Leave in a large jar in the airing cupboard, or similar warm dark place, and rinse twice daily. In a few days they will have sprouted, and are delicious to eat. Also experiment with beans and seeds.	Go for a long walk in the country or a park. Have a picnic if the weather is good.

DAY	DIET TIP (Add the day's tip to all the previous days' tips)	DAILY SELF-INVESTMENT TIP
23	Make up a new recipe using coconut milk, vegetables and brown rice.	This is your chance to try your hand at an old hobby, such as sport, painting or drawing. Spend the whole day at it, and if you enjoy it, resolve to continue.
24	From now until the end of the month, make yourself a daily energizing and cleansing juice or smoothie.	Work on the Win/Win model (see page 24).
25	Eat a salad with your meal, with a tahini, lemon juice and garlic dressing.	Work on the exercise on immediate gratification in "I want it now!" on page 26.
26	Eat a new fruit. Get some ideas from "Stress-busting superfoods" on page 74.	Work out some time-management improvements you can make in your life.
27	CLEANSING DAY. Eat fruit and vegetables only, and drink water (hot or cold).	Treat yourself to a professional massage.
28	As well as fruit and vegetables, eat some protein such as tofu, beans, a little fish or organic chicken.	Focus on "Positive self-talk" (page 149).
29	Enjoy a meal out. Choose a dish that contains no wheat, dairy products or sugar.	Today is a day of relaxation – enjoy it! Go for a stroll. Apply a face pack and give yourself a manicure.
30	Tomorrow you can start to reintroduce foods you have been avoiding, such as wheat. Reintroduce them, one per day, every two or three days over the next week. Make a note of any adverse reactions and avoid foods that do not agree with you.	Skin brush and have a long sea-salt bath with candles and soft music. Wrap yourself in a warm towel, massage yourself with almond oil and go to bed early.

Congratulations, you've done it! Remember to keep your diet varied from now on. If you include sugar, alcohol, tea and coffee in your diet again, keep them to an absolute minimum and do not slip back into old ways.

Nothing comes from nothing.

WILLIAM SHAKESPEARE

IDENTIFYING FOOD SENSITIVITIES

Your one-month plan is a good opportunity to find out whether you are sensitive to any foods. The most common allergens are wheat and dairy products, but any food may cause problems to a particular individual.

Common signs of allergy include digestive disturbances such as bloating, flatulence, indigestion and irritable bowel syndrome, as well as a range of other symptoms including headaches, skin problems, arthritis, mood swings and PMS.

ALTERNATIVES TO WHEAT

Wheat products include bread, pasta, cous-cous, wheat crackers, pastry, biscuits, semolina, bulgar wheat, wheat cereal, puffed wheat.
- Rye. Crackers, bread, pumpernickel bread.
- Oats. Porridge, oatcakes, flapjacks.
- Barley. Cook it like rice.
- Corn. Corn bread, popcorn, nachos, pasta, polenta.
- Millet. Porridge, flakes, cook it like rice.
- Rice. Pasta, noodles, rice cakes, puffed rice.
- Quinoa. Cooked like rice.
- Buckwheat. Noodles, kasha, pasta.

N.B. Although bulgar is cracked wheat (a type of wheat), it is often tolerated by those who cannot have other wheat products.

The one-month plan stipulates the avoidance of wheat, dairy products, sugar, tea and coffee. If you suspect you have an allergy or sensitivity to any other food, cut it out during the month as well. To test suspect foods, avoid them for two weeks and then reintroduce them one at a time, monitoring symptoms that occur.

SCALP MASSAGE

An Indian head massage is one of the most relaxing ways to unwind. You can do it yourself, or even better, ask someone to do it for you.

You will need about three tablespoonsful of almond oil or jojoba oil. Part your hair at intervals and rub the oil into your scalp with a cotton wool ball. Make sure you cover the whole of your head, including the back. Using your fingertips, and applying firm pressure, massage your scalp. Pour any remaining oil onto the rest of your hair. Wrap your head in a towel and leave the oil on for a couple of hours, or even overnight (place another towel over your pillow). You will need two good lathers when you wash it to remove the oil.

TIME MANAGEMENT

One of the main causes of stress is is not having enough time to do all the things you want to do. Here are some tips on time management to incorporate into your day.

- Set priorities.
- Tackle tough jobs first.
- Use it, file it, bin it.
- Delegate.
- Allow sufficient time for travelling.
- Realize that all jobs take longer than you think they will.
- Don't be a perfectionist.
- At the end of each day, set your agenda for the next.

ALTERNATIVES TO DAIRY PRODUCTS

Dairy products include milk, yoghurt and cheese.

■ Soya milk, soya yoghurt, soya cheese, tofu.

■ Rice milk.

■ Oat milk or oat fibre yoghurt.

■ Coconut cream.

■ Nut milks (almonds and other nuts can be used).

N.B. Some people find that although they cannot tolerate cow's milk, they are able to eat cow's milk yoghurt, also goat's and sheep's milk and their products. Butter is 100 per cent fat and so is rarely a source of dairy intolerance.

EXPAND YOUR HORIZONS

This month may also be a good time for you to stretch yourself by taking on a new challenge. By doing this, you increase your command over your life. We all conduct our lives at a level that we feel comfortable with, but sometimes this leads us to get stuck in a routine that cuts out a world of wonderful possibilities.

For your challenge, choose something that you have wanted to do for a while. You may want to expand your social life by inviting round people you would not normally have the courage to ask. You could sign up for a course in something you felt too timid to try before. You could read a book that challenges you intellectually.

POSITIVE SELF-TALK

It is very easy to berate yourself when things do not go according to plan: "Oh my goodness, you are so stupid", "How could you do that?", "Don't you ever think?", "I really can't believe you said something so dumb".

If your partner, friend, or boss spoke to you like this, the chances are that you would storm off in a huff. But how many times a day do you talk to yourself in this way? Why do you accept these damaging, demoralizing and stressful words from yourself, when you would not dream of taking them from others? Do not underestimate how upsetting this kind of communication can be – it reinforces negative images and perpetuates low self-esteem.

Carry a notebook with you for a couple of weeks and write down every time you speak to yourself in this way. Write down even the smallest reproach. Read through the resulting collection of admonitions, and see if you can think of more appropriate language to use. This does not mean saying inanely, "I love and respect myself" 20 times a day, but finding a middle ground between the difficulty of a situation and a constructive way of responding to it.

At first, you may feel awkward. But persevere and you will find that communicating with yourself – the most important person in your life – improves beyond measure. And yes, you will learn to love and respect yourself!

WE'RE ALL GOING ON A SUMMER HOLIDAY

It is often difficult to set aside time for yourself. The busiest people quite often do not take their full holiday entitlement from work, but this does not do their employers any favours, because even the most motivated workers gradually become more run down and less focused. Everybody needs a break.

● Get out your diary right now. Plan at least one reasonable break every four months.

● If your experience of previous holidays has been that you feel more exhausted when you get back, work out what needs to change in order to improve matters. Do you do too much of your own catering? Do you need to find more for the kids to do? Do you end up doing what your partner wants to do, instead of what you want to do?

● You are at the airport, ready for a relaxing break, and you buy a novel for the journey, described as "Mystery. Murder. Intrigue. Gripping suspense". After a couple of hours of high-adrenaline reading on the beach, you are ready for a little surfing or water-skiing, something to get the adrenaline going again. Are you addicted to stress? Do you really want to unwind on holiday?

● Research has shown that short breaks are not as restful as longer breaks. Some of the time is lost in travelling, and there isn't long enough to fully unwind. Take at least one, and preferably two, two-week holidays a year.

● More than a third of people use their annual holiday as a time to plan their lives, deciding to change jobs, move house or to carry out major renovations. A holiday may be the only time you have to stop and think, but resolve to set aside time during the year for these planning exercises, so that you can really enjoy your vacations.

INSTEAD OF	SAY TO YOURSELF
That was so stupid!	My reaction did not serve me well, but next time I will do better.
Why do I always mess things up?	I can't get it right all the time, and I can aim to do better next time.
I'm so slow!	I need time to achieve the results I am seeking.
Why do I waste my time so much?	Nothing is a waste of time. I always learn something. I can be more selective in future.
I'm so disorganized.	My organizational skills need working on.

DAILY STRESS BUSTERS

Try these strategies for keeping stress at bay – if you practise them every day, they will help you in the long run.

● Laugh! Laughing raises endorphins, the feel-good hormones, and strengthens the immune system. A laugh a day keeps the doctor away.

● Put your daily problems in perspective. Don't let things niggle you. Work out if they are really important or if you are over-reacting – the only person to suffer will be you.

● Dilute a few drops of a calming essential oil in a carrier oil and dab it behind

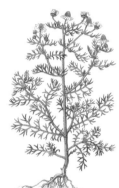

your ears, or drop on to a cotton-wool ball kept in a pot on your desk. Ylang-ylang, chamomile, lavender or neroli will have the desired effect.

● Take it easy. Don't rush. It doesn't matter if you miss that train or bus – another will come along. Get up a little earlier to avoid a frenzied start to the day. Prepare well ahead for deadlines.

● Don't be a perfectionist. Do enough to make something work, but don't overdo it.

● Doodle or find some other mindless pursuit to occupy a quarter of an hour. Constant concentration can burn you out. Sing or hum to relieve tension.

● Surround yourself with cool, calming colours such as blue, purple and green (on cushions, flowers, desk items) to create a relaxing environment.

● Eat slowly and chew thoroughly.

MEDITATION

Meditation has been practised for over 4,000 years and is mentioned in the Vedas, the sacred writings of Hinduism. Meditation is an integral part of yoga, and has been found to heal the body on many levels – physical, mental and spiritual.

● Meditation helps to deal with stress and is excellent for reducing anxiety.

● It helps to modify the suppressive effect strenuous physical exercise has on immune function.

● It aids recovery from addictions.

● It significantly improves blood fat levels, and can assist those convalescing from heart disease.

● It improves the balance between cortisol and DHEA. These hormones are often out of balance in people under long-term stress.

● Insomnia can be eradicated by using meditation.

Find out about meditation courses in your area. If there are none, a course in Autogenic Therapy, Psychocalisthenics™ or Tai Chi would be a good alternative.

Growth is the only evidence of life.

JOHN HENRY NEWMAN

Useful addresses

Institute For Optimum Nutrition
Blades Court
Deodar Road
London SW15 2NU
Tel: 020 8877 9993

**Society For The Promotion Of
Nutritional Therapy**
P.O. Box 626
Woking
Surrey GU22 0XD
Tel: 01483 740 903

**Association of Systematic Kinesiology
(Muscle testing)**
39 Browns Road
Surbiton
Surrey KT5 8ST
Tel: 020 8399 3215

British Herbal Medicine Association
P.O. Box 304
Bournemouth
BH7 6JZ
Tel: 01202 433691

Simply Organic
Home delivery of organic foods
Tel: 0845 1000 444
www.simplyorganic.net

American Association of World Health
1129-2012 st, NW, ste. 400
Washington DC 20036 3403
USA

National Institute of Nutritional Education
1010 s. Jolier St
Aurora, CO 80012
USA

Useful websites

Austin Nutritional Research
www.realtime.net/anr/
Food and Nutrition Internet Navigator
www.fnii.ifis.org
Tufts University Nutrition Navigator
www.navigator.tufts.ed

For information on Suzannah Olivier's
activities visit her website:
healthandnutrition.co.uk
or email eattobefit@aol.com

OTHER SITES:
www.positivehealth.com
www.healthy.net
www.thinknatural.com
www.livingfoods.enta.net
www.realhealth.co.uk
www.glutenfree-foods.co.uk

Further reading

Cooking Without
Barbara Cousins
(Harper Collins, 1997)

Super Juice
Michael Van Straten
(Mitchell Beazley, 1999)

Seasonal Affective Disorder
Angela Smith
(Thorsons, 1991)

Optimum Nutrition Cookbook
Patrick Holford and Judy Ridgeway
(Piatkus, 1999)

Maximising Energy
Suzannah Olivier
(Simon and Schuster, 2000)

Juice and Zest
Anna Selby
(Collins and Brown, 2000)

Herbal and nutrient supplement supplies

Biocare
Tel: 0121 433 3727

Higher Nature
Tel: 01435 882880

Lamberts
Tel: 01892 552120

The Nutri Centre
Tel: 020 7436 5122

Solgar
Tel: 01442 890355
www.solgar.com

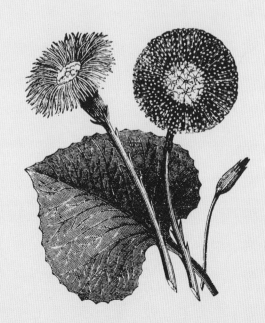

Index

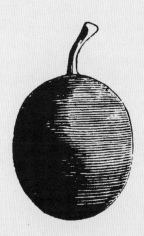

Acknowledgements

With thanks to Ruth Katz for introducing me to Liz; Liz Dean for having the vision; Carol Heaton for all her hard work on my behalf; Fiona Jenkins for her insight, common sense and superb work; and, as ever, Laurence for putting up with me tapping on the keyboard at all hours.

PICTURE CREDITS

Cover: Collins & Brown

P7 Pictor International; **p8-9** C&B; **p11** The Ronald Grant Archive; **p13** C&B; **p15** Gettyone Stone; **p19** Gettyone Stone; **p20** Allsport/Hulton Deutsch; **p23** right & bottom left Telegraph Colour Library, top left Rita Maas/The Image Bank; **p24** Morrell/The Image Bank; **P25** Saturday Evening Post/The Advertising Archives; **p26** Telegraph Colour Library; **p27** UIP/The Ronald Grant Archive; **p29 & 31** Gettyone Stone; **p32-33** C&B; **p35** Bob Elsdale/The Image Bank; **p37** left Telegraph Colour Library, right Britt Erlanson/The Image Bank; **p38** The Ronald Grant Archive; **p42**

& 43 C&B; **p44** Gettyone Stone; **p45** Telegraph Colour Library; **p48** The Kobal Collection; **p50** The Telegraph Colour Library; **p52** C&B; **p53** bottom right Jacqui Hurst, rest C&B; **p54** Phototake NYC/Robert Harding.com; **p56-57** C&B; **p58, 61, 65, 67, 68, 69, 71 & 73** C&B; **p69** right The Anthony Blake Photo Library; **p74** centre right Gettyone Stone, rest C&B; **p75** centre Pictor International, right Gettyone Stone, rest C&B; **p76** right Gettyone Stone, rest C&B; **p77** left The Anthony Blake Photo Library, centre right GPL/Joanne Pavia, right The Anthony Blake Photo Library copyright Martin Brigdale, rest C&B; **p78** centre right & right Telegraph Colour Library, rest C&B; **p79** centre left & centre Gettyone Stone, centre right Telegraph Colour

Library, rest C&B; **p80** left & bottom right Gettyone Stone, top right C&B; **p81 & 82** C&B; **p83** top C&B, bottom Pictor International; **p85, 87, 88, 89 & 91** C&B; **p92** top right Telegraph Colour Library, rest C&B; **p93, 94 & 95** C&B; **p97** bottom left Gettyone Stone, rest C&B; **p98** Pictor International; **p99** Telegraph Colour Library; **p101** Gettyone Stone; **p109** Telegraph Colour Library; **p110-111** C&B; **p114 & 115** C&B; **p117** Gettyone Stone; **p118** Telegraph Colour Library; **p119** C&B; **p125** Gettyone Stone; **p126** Pictor International; **p127 & 129** C&B; **p131** Gettyone Stone; **p133, 135 & 136** C&B; **p137** Gettyone Stone; **p139** top C&B, bottom Antonio Rosario/The Image Bank; **p140** top C&B, bottom Pictor International; **p141 & 143** Gettyone Stone; **p149, 151** C&B